Pulmonary Metastasectomy

Editors

MARK W. ONAITIS
THOMAS A. D'AMICO

THORACIC
SURGERY CLINICS

www.thoracic.theclinics.com

Consulting Editor
M. BLAIR MARSHALL

February 2016 • Volume 26 • Number 1

ELSEVIER

1600 John F. Kennedy Boulevard • Suite 1800 • Philadelphia, Pennsylvania, 19103-2899

http://www.thoracic.theclinics.com

THORACIC SURGERY CLINICS Volume 26, Number 1
February 2016 ISSN 1547-4127, ISBN-13: 978-0-323-41716-7

Editor: John Vassallo (j.vassallo@elsevier.com)
Developmental Editor: Susan Showalter

Thoracic Surgery Clinics (ISSN 1547-4127) is published quarterly by Elsevier Inc., 360 Park Avenue South, New York, NY 10010-1710. Months of publication are February, May, August, and November. Business and editorial offices: 1600 John F. Kennedy Boulevard, Suite 1800, Philadelphia, PA 19103-2899. Periodicals postage paid at New York, NY, and additional mailing offices. Subscription prices are $355.00 per year (US individuals), $501.00 per year (US institutions), $100.00 per year (US Students), $435.00 per year (Canadian individuals), $648.00 per year (Canadian institutions), $225.00 per year (Canadian and international students), $465.00 per year (international individuals), and $648.00 per year (international institutions). Foreign air speed delivery is included in all Clinics' subscription prices. All prices are subject to change without notice. **POSTMASTER:** Send address changes to Thoracic Surgery Clinics, Elsevier Health Sciences Division, Subscription Customer Service, 3251 Riverport Lane, Maryland Heights, MO 63043. **Customer Service (orders, claims, online, change of address): Telephone: 1-800-654-2452 (U.S. and Canada); 314-447-8871 (outside U.S. and Canada). Fax: 314-447-8029. E-mail: journalscustomerservice-usa@elsevier.com (for print support); journalsonlinesupport-usa@elsevier.com (for online support).**

Reprints. For copies of 100 or more, of articles in this publication, please contact Commercial Rights Department, Elsevier Inc., 360 Park Avenue South, New York, NY 10010-1710. Tel: 212-633-3874; Fax: 212-633-3820; E-mail: reprints@elsevier.com.

Thoracic Surgery Clinics is covered in *MEDLINE/PubMed (Index Medicus), EMBASE/Excerpta Medica, Science Citation Index Expanded (SciSearch®), Journal Citation Reports/Science Edition,* and *Current Contents®/Clinical Medicine.*

Contributors

CONSULTING EDITOR

M. BLAIR MARSHALL, MD, FACS
Chief, Division of Thoracic Surgery; Associate
Professor of Surgery, Department of Surgery,
Georgetown University Medical Center,
Georgetown University School of Medicine,
Washington, DC

EDITORS

MARK W. ONAITIS, MD
Associate Professor of Surgery, Section of
General Thoracic Surgery, Department of
Surgery, Duke University Medical Center,
Durham, North Carolina

THOMAS A. D'AMICO, MD
Gary Hock Endowed Professor of Surgery,
Chief, Section of General Thoracic Surgery;
Program Director, Thoracic Surgery, Duke
University Medical Center, Durham,
North Carolina

AUTHORS

MANJIT S. BAINS, MD
Professor of Surgery, Thoracic Service,
Department of Surgery, Memorial Hospital,
Memorial Sloan-Kettering Cancer Center,
New York, New York

DAVID BALL, MB BS, MD, FRANZCR
Department of Radiation Oncology, Peter
MacCallum Cancer Centre, Melbourne,
Victoria, Australia; The Sir Peter MacCallum
Department of Oncology, The University of
Melbourne, Parkville, Victoria, Australia

SHANDA H. BLACKMON, MD, MPH
Associate Professor of Thoracic Surgery,
Division of General Thoracic Surgery, Mayo
Clinic, Rochester, Minnesota

MATTHEW J. BOYER, MD, PhD
Department of Radiation Oncology, Duke
University, Durham, North Carolina

DUYKHANH P. CEPPA, MD
Assistant Professor of Surgery, Division of
Cardiothoracic Surgery, Department of
Surgery, Indiana University School of
Medicine, Indianapolis, Indiana

TODD L. DEMMY, MD
Chair, Thoracic Surgery, Professor of
Oncology, Roswell Park Cancer Institute,
Professor of Surgery, State University of New
York at Buffalo, Buffalo, New York

**KAREN J. DICKINSON, MBBS, BSc, MD,
FRCS**
Division of General Thoracic Surgery, Mayo
Clinic, Rochester, Minnesota

ROBERT J. DOWNEY, MD
Professor of Surgery, Thoracic Service,
Department of Surgery, Memorial Hospital,
Memorial Sloan-Kettering Cancer Center,
New York, New York

LORETTA ERHUNMWUNSEE, MD
Assistant Professor, Division of Thoracic
Surgery, City of Hope Comprehensive Cancer
Center, Duarte, California

DAVID H. HARPOLE, MD
Professor of Surgery; Associate Professor of
Pathology, Duke University, Durham, North
Carolina

ELISABETH KNÖCHLEIN, MD
Department of Thoracic Surgery, Dr Horst
Schmidt Klinik, Wiesbaden, Germany

NATALIE KUDELIN, MD
Department of Thoracic Surgery, Dr Horst
Schmidt Klinik, Wiesbaden, Germany

FERGUS MACBETH, MA, DM, FRCR, FRCP
Wales Cancer Trials Unit, University Hospital of
Wales, Heath Park, Cardiff, United Kingdom

MICHAEL A. MORSE, MD, MHS
Professor of Medicine, Division of Medical
Oncology, Duke University Medical Center,
Durham, North Carolina

HARVEY PASS, MD
Stephen E. Banner Professor of Thoracic
Oncology, Vice-Chair Research, Department of
Cardiothoracic Surgery, Division Chief,
General Thoracic Surgery, NYU Langone
Medical Center, New York, New York

KIRILL PROKRYM, BA
Department of Cardiothoracic Surgery, NYU
Langone Medical Center, New York, New York

JAMES MATTHEW REINERSMAN, MD
Assistant Professor, Division of Thoracic &
Cardiovascular Surgery, Department of
Surgery, University of Oklahoma Health
Sciences Center, Oklahoma City, Oklahoma

UMBERTO RICARDI, MD
Department of Oncology, University of Turin,
Turin, Italy

JOSEPH K. SALAMA, MD
Department of Radiation Oncology, Duke
University, Durham, North Carolina

JOACHIM SCHIRREN, MD
Department of Thoracic Surgery, Dr Horst
Schmidt Klinik, Wiesbaden, Germany

MORITZ SCHIRREN, MD
Department of Thoracic Surgery, Dr Horst
Schmidt Klinik, Wiesbaden, Germany

CHRISTOPHER D. SCOTT, MD
Cardiothoracic Resident, Department of
Surgery, Duke University, Duke University
Medical Center, Durham, North Carolina

ELLIOT SERVAIS, MD
Chief Resident, Cardiothoracic Surgery,
Brigham and Women's Hospital,
Harvard Medical School, Boston,
Massachusetts

STEFAN SPONHOLZ, MD
Department of Thoracic Surgery, Dr Horst
Schmidt Klinik, Wiesbaden, Germany

SCOTT J. SWANSON, MD
Director, Minimally Invasive Thoracic
Surgery; Vice Chair, Cancer Affairs,
Department of Surgery, Chief Surgical Officer,
Dana-Farber Cancer Institute, Brigham and
Women's Hospital, Professor of Surgery,
Harvard Medical School, Boston,
Massachusetts

BETTY C. TONG, MD, MHS
Associate Professor, Division of
Cardiovascular and Thoracic Surgery,
Department of Surgery, Duke
University Medical Center, Durham,
North Carolina

TOM TREASURE, MD, MS, FRCS, FRCP
Clinical Operational Research Unit, University
College London, London, United Kingdom

ALISON WARD, MD
Department of Cardiothoracic Surgery, NYU
Langone Medical Center, New York, New York

DENNIS A. WIGLE, MD, PhD
Associate Professor, Division of General
Thoracic Surgery, Department of Surgery,
Mayo Clinic, Rochester, Minnesota

Contents

Preface: Modern Management of Pulmonary Metastases xi

Mark W. Onaitis and Thomas A. D'Amico

The Biology of Pulmonary Metastasis 1

Christopher D. Scott and David H. Harpole

The process of metastasis relies on a series of stochastic and sequential steps, with selective pressure exerted on a large number of genetically volatile cancer cells to produce a very small fraction of tumor cells with the ability to navigate the transition from primary tumor cell to end-organ metastasis. This process is intricately determined by cell-microenvironment interactions, the mechanistic understanding of which is steadily increasing. The continued elucidation of pathways that govern these interactions offers potential therapeutic options to patients with advanced disease.

Preoperative Evaluation and Indications for Pulmonary Metastasectomy 7

Loretta Erhunmwunsee and Betty C. Tong

Most patients with pulmonary metastases will not be candidates for pulmonary metastasectomy. Preoperative evaluation determines whether a patient is both fit enough for surgery and has disease that is actually resectable. Both components are necessary for patients who undergo resection with curative intent. In general, to be considered for pulmonary metastasectomy, patients must fit the following criteria: the primary disease site and any extrathoracic disease are both controlled; complete resection of pulmonary involvement is achievable with adequate pulmonary reserve; and there are no effective medical therapies.

Open Surgical Approaches for Pulmonary Metastasectomy 13

Robert J. Downey and Manjit S. Bains

Surgeons differ in the approach to resection of pulmonary metastases from nonpulmonary primary malignancies, with some favoring procedures that minimize trauma to the patient, and others performing open procedures with the goal of maximizing likelihood of resection of all detectable sites of disease. This article reviews how pulmonary metastasectomy emerged as a therapy for metastatic disease. Discussed is how surgical approaches used for this procedure have evolved, the available literature addressing whether open procedures lead to more complete resections, and if so whether resection by open procedures increases the likelihood of cure following resection. The technical aspects of the various thoracotomy techniques are also reviewed.

Ablative Approaches for Pulmonary Metastases 19

Matthew J. Boyer, Umberto Ricardi, David Ball, and Joseph K. Salama

Pulmonary metastases are common in patients with cancer for which surgery is considered a standard approach in appropriately selected patients. A number of patients are not candidates for surgery due to a medical comorbidities or the extent of surgery required. For these patients, noninvasive or minimally invasive approaches to ablate pulmonary metastases are potential treatment strategies. This article summarizes the rationale and outcomes for non-surgical treatment approaches, including radiotherapy, radiofrequency and microwave ablation, for pulmonary metastases.

Lymphadenectomy During Pulmonary Metastasectomy   35

James Matthew Reinersman and Dennis A. Wigle

Pulmonary metastasectomy continues to be an effective approach to prolong survival in appropriately selected patients. The incidence of lymphatic spread is more common than previously recognized, with an estimate of 20% to 25% across multiple tumor types. The presence of metastatically involved lymph nodes adversely affects survival. What remains unclear is whether N1 vs N2, or the number of stations involved affects survival differently. The role of surgery for pulmonary metastasectomy in the patient with nodal metastases will likely expand with ongoing improvements in targeted and immunotherapies.

Results of Pulmonary Resection: Colorectal Carcinoma   41

Karen J. Dickinson and Shanda H. Blackmon

Whether pulmonary metastasectomy improves survival in patients with metastatic colorectal cancer is controversial. Wedge resection is the most common form of surgical intervention. When anatomic resection is required, segmentectomy may be preferable to lobectomy for preservation of lung parenchyma. Each intervention to remove metastatic pulmonary parenchymal disease should consider future disease recurrence. Nonoperative modalities, such as radiofrequency ablation, cryoablation, and microwave ablation, are becoming more popular regarding parenchymal preservation. The future may embrace complex risk-profile analysis including molecular markers, nomograms to predict survival, and hybrid treatment approaches. Minimally invasive surgical techniques are used with increased frequency, making reoperative metastasectomy less tedious.

Results of Pulmonary Resection: Sarcoma and Germ Cell Tumors   49

DuyKhanh P. Ceppa

Pulmonary metastasis occurs in as many as 88% and 80% of stage IV patients with sarcoma and germ cell tumors, respectively. Pulmonary metastatectomy may be the only means of rendering a patient disease free. Sublobar resection (wedge or segmentectomy), lobectomy, and pneumonectomy achieve complete resection. Bilateral disease can be resected via staged thoracoscopy/thoracotomy, median sternotomy, or clamshell thoracotomy. Multiple resections and re-resections have resulted in improved survival. Five-year survival rates as high as 35% to 52% for sarcoma and 80% for germ cell tumor can be realized.

Isolated Lung Perfusion for Pulmonary Metastases   55

Alison Ward, Kirill Prokrym, and Harvey Pass

Isolated lung perfusion (ILP) is a surgical technique developed to treat pulmonary metastases. During ILP, high-dose chemotherapy is delivered into the pulmonary vasculature, minimizing systemic exposure and delivering the chemotherapeutic agent directly to the lung. ILP has been studied extensively in a variety of animal models and in humans in phase I trials. The most frequently studied chemotherapeutic agents used in ILP are doxorubicin, 5-flurodeoxyuridine, tumor necrosis factor-α, paclitaxel, melphalan, gemcitabine, and cisplatin. Phase I clinical trials with ILP have shown that ILP can be safely performed in humans but with mixed clinical results and poor long-term survival.

Immunotherapy for Resected Pulmonary Metastases 69

Michael A. Morse

Micrometastatic disease following pulmonary metastasectomy is an ideal setting to test adjuvant immunotherapy, as the efficacy of immunotherapy in experimental models is greatest with the smallest tumor burdens. Although there is not a standard-of-care adjuvant immunotherapy for resected pulmonary metastases, there have been several studies using cytokines and other immunostimulatory molecules in conjunction with metastasectomies in patients with melanoma, renal cell carcinoma, sarcoma, and colorectal cancer, which have provided preliminary data that such adjuvant therapy is feasible and safe and may be useful in the future, following more rigorous testing, as routine therapy to prevent recurrences.

Is Surgery Warranted for Oligometastatic Disease? 79

Tom Treasure and Fergus Macbeth

The development of metastases after curative treatment can be seen as a failure. A common justification for the removal of metastases is that the knowledge that they are there may cause psychological distress, a real symptom that may be relieved by their removal. Although it is a commonly used justification for metastasectomy, the authors are unaware of any studies confirming or quantifying the health gain. This article strongly challenges the belief in clinical effectiveness and demonstrates that it is supported neither by a sound biological rationale nor by any good evidence. Reasons are suggested why this unfounded belief has become so prevalent.

Thoracoscopic Management of Pulmonary Metastases 91

Elliot Servais and Scott J. Swanson

In appropriately selected patients, resection of pulmonary metastases from various primary tumors can lead to improved survival. Metastasectomy has traditionally been performed by open thoracotomy; however, thoracoscopic resection offers the important benefits of a less invasive approach with more expeditious recovery. Concerns regarding missed lesions during thoracoscopy have not been realized in analyses of survival and may be offset by a policy of repeat metastasectomy for pulmonary recurrences. Despite the relative paucity of prospective trials, the preponderance of data supports the use of video-assisted thoracic surgery for pulmonary metastasectomy, which represents our preferred strategy for these patients.

Results of Pulmonary Resection: Other Epithelial Malignancies 99

Stefan Sponholz, Moritz Schirren, Natalie Kudelin, Elisabeth Knöchlein, and Joachim Schirren

This article summarizes the interdisciplinary work, survival, prognostic factors, and prognostic groups for lung metastases from breast cancer and renal cell cancer. Furthermore, the prevalence of lymph node metastases and the importance of a systematic lymph node dissection in metastasectomy of breast cancer and renal cell cancer for a true R0 resection are discussed.

Thoracoscopic Lung Suffusion   **109**

Todd L. Demmy

 Videos of basic setup and vein isolation, retrograde suffusion flow, and the suffusion sequence accompany this article

The lung is a common site of metastatic disease, which may be the only measurable malignancy in some patients. Unfortunately, because of the invasiveness of previous techniques and the fragility of these target organs, many attempts at regional lung therapies have not become that popular. Accordingly, a method for thoracoscopic vascular control to enable permeation of the lung with agents was developed and termed *suffusion* to distinguish it from earlier methods. This article describes the preclinical work supporting lung suffusion and our early human experience.

Index   **123**

THORACIC SURGERY CLINICS

FORTHCOMING ISSUES

May 2016
Innovations in Thoracic Surgery
Kazuhiro Yasufuku, *Editor*

August 2016
Supportive Evidence in Thoracic Surgery
Michael Lanuti, *Editor*

November 2016
Management of Hyperhidrosis
Peter B. Licht, *Editor*

RECENT ISSUES

November 2015
Prevention and Management of Postoperative Complications
John D. Mitchell, *Editor*

August 2015
Management of Intraoperative Crises
Shanda H. Blackmon, *Editor*

May 2015
Lung Cancer Screening
Gaetano Rocco, *Editor*

RELATED INTEREST

Surgical Clinics, Volume 95, Issue 5 (October 2015)
Cancer Screening and Genetics
Christopher L. Wolfgang, *Editor*
Available at: www.surgical.theclinics.com

THE CLINICS ARE AVAILABLE ONLINE!
Access your subscription at:
www.theclinics.com

Preface
Modern Management of Pulmonary Metastases

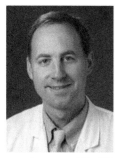 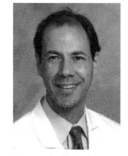

Mark W. Onaitis, MD   Thomas A. D'Amico, MD

Editors

The management of pulmonary metastases has evolved considerably over the last several decades, yet is still a controversial issue, in part due to the lack of prospective data regarding operative and nonoperative management. In this issue of *Thoracic Surgery Clinics*, we offer a comprehensive, well-organized, and state-of-the-art synopsis of the essential topics regarding the management of pulmonary metastases, including options for local therapy, conventional systemic therapy, immunologic therapy, and isolated perfusion strategies.

Understanding the biology of pulmonary metastases is essential to understanding the options for treatment. The role of surgery is debated articulately, and this argument sheds light on the importance of patient selection, among other important principles. The role of open versus minimally invasive surgical approaches is also analyzed, including the trends that favor the thoracoscopic approach. Local control with surgery is currently being challenged by the various options of ablative therapies.

While the management of pulmonary metastases is founded on these fundamental concepts, individual patient management is also influenced by the primary histology, and the management of the most common histologies is also reviewed: colorectal cancer and other epithelial malignancies, sarcoma, and germ cell tumors. Finally, the innovative approaches of isolated pulmonary suffusion and perfusion are discussed.

With the development of more effective systemic therapy for metastatic disease, it is probable that more patients will be considered candidates for management of pulmonary metastases. A thorough understanding of the biology, evaluation, and options for treatment are essential in order to achieve the best outcomes.

Mark W. Onaitis, MD
Duke University Medical Center
DUMC Box 3305
Durham, NC 27710, USA

Thomas A. D'Amico, MD
Duke University Medical Center
DUMC Box 3496
Duke South, White Zone
Room 3589
Durham, NC 27710, USA

E-mail addresses:
mark.onaitis@dm.duke.edu (M.W. Onaitis)
thomas.damico@duke.edu (T.A. D'Amico)

Thorac Surg Clin 26 (2016) xi
http://dx.doi.org/10.1016/j.thorsurg.2015.10.001
1547-4127/16/$ – see front matter © 2016 Published by Elsevier Inc.

The Biology of Pulmonary Metastasis

Christopher D. Scott, MD[a], David H. Harpole, MD[b],*

KEYWORDS

- Metastasis • Pulmonary metastasis • Seed and soil hypothesis

KEY POINTS

- The process of metastasis relies on a series of stochastic and sequential steps, with selective pressure exerted on a large number of genetically volatile cancer cells to produce a very small fraction of tumor cells with the ability to navigate the transition from primary tumor cell to end-organ metastasis.
- Metastasis is intricately determined by cell-microenvironment interactions, of which we are steadily gaining a mechanistic understanding.
- The continued elucidation of pathways that govern these interactions offers potential therapeutic options to patients with advanced disease.

INTRODUCTION

The study of cancer metastasis has been a process spanning nearly 2 centuries, and only over the few decades have we begun to mechanistically break down the complex interactions that influence a transformed cell to progress to metastasis. Investigations from recent literature have demonstrated that from the potentially millions of cancer cells shed into the circulation, only a minute fraction of these cells have the capability of forming metastasis in distant organs. This process is not governed simply by the volume of exposure to an organ, but is marked by stochastic intrinsic cellular events and is influenced by selective evolutionary pressure exerted on the cell by its local environment. This process was elegantly described more than 100 years ago by Stephen Paget, who published his enduring article on the "seed and soil" hypothesis to explain the nonrandom pattern of metastasis.[1] He observed a discrepancy between the blood supply and frequency of metastasis to distant organs based on autopsy records from 735 women with breast cancer. He posited that "remote organs cannot be altogether passive or indifferent regarding [tumor] embolism."

The biological cascade of events required for cancer metastasis includes increased motility, loss of cellular adhesions, intravasation to the circulation, survival while in transit, extravasation to distant organs, and colonization. Each step in the process is necessary, and failure of any these can prove to be rate limiting. Clinicians have become increasingly aware of the various genes and pathways that regulate these interactions between tumor cell and host. As research continues to elucidate the biology of cancer metastasis and identify molecular pathways and mediators we can begin to more accurately determine molecular signatures that serve as surrogate markers for a metastatic phenotype. Furthermore, as the understanding of the mechanistic processes of cell and microenvironment interactions increases, therapeutic interventions can be developed to target specific stages in the progression of a cancer cell to a metastasis.

AN OVERVIEW OF THE PATHOGENESIS OF METASTASIS

The cascade of cancer metastasis consists of a sequential and interrelated series of steps, each

[a] Department of Surgery, Duke University, Duke University Medical Center, 4. DUMC Box 3627, Durham, NC 27710, USA; [b] Duke University, Durham, NC 27710, USA
* Corresponding author.
E-mail address: david.harpole@dm.duke.edu

Thorac Surg Clin 26 (2016) 1–6
http://dx.doi.org/10.1016/j.thorsurg.2015.09.001
1547-4127/16/$ – see front matter © 2016 Elsevier Inc. All rights reserved.

of which can be rate limiting.[2] The progression to metastasis involves establishing neovasculature,[3] altered cellular adhesion,[4] increased cell motility,[5] disruption of the basement membrane,[6,7] intravasation to the circulation,[2,8] escaping host immune surveillance,[9] tumor embolization, and arrest in capillary beds and eventual colonization of a distant site.[10,11] As outlined in the seed and soil hypothesis,[1] the interaction between host and cell factors determines which organs can support the survival of metastasis.

The Heterogeneity of Metastasis

It has been well demonstrated that not all cells located in the primary tumor have a similar potential to metastasis. Prior experiments have demonstrated that cells with differing metastatic potential have been isolated from the same parent tumor[12] and that highly metastatic clones from tumor cell populations demonstrate a higher rate of genetic mutability than nonmetastatic clones from the same tumor.[13] Heterogeneity within a population is a requirement of any evolutionary process, and allows a source of advantageous traits from which to select from. When applied to the biology of metastasis, several factors contribute to the instability of the cancer genome: DNA mutations, chromosomal arrangements, and epigenetic alterations.[14] Several mutations have been proposed that cause genomic instability and lead to tumor proliferation. Inactivation of cell-cycle suppressors,[15] disabling DNA-damage sensors,[16] and telomeric crisis[17] are a few of the putative pathways. Epigenetic plasticity also plays a significant role in metastatic heterogeneity.[18,19]

The Clonality of Metastasis

Previous animal experiments have demonstrated that tumor progression is associated with increasing genetic instability and spontaneous mutation rates,[13] supporting the hypothesis that acquired genetic variability within developing clones of tumors, coupled with selection pressures, results in the emergence of tumor cell variants with increasing malignant potential.[20] To determine the clonality of cancer metastasis, Talmadge and colleagues[21] conducted a series of experiments in which random chromosome breaks were used as unique indelible markers. The metastatic phenotypes of spontaneous lung metastases derived from subcutaneously implanted tumors were analyzed whereby unique karyotypic patterns of abnormal marker chromosomes were identified, indicating that the metastases had originated from a single progenitor cell.

Several other reports have demonstrated the clonality of other tumors in melanoma, breast, and fibrosarcoma.[22]

SEED AND SOIL, REVISITED

In 1889, Stephen Paget was the first to address the question, "What is it that decides what organs shall suffer in a case of disseminated cancer?"[1] In doing so he established the framework for tumor-cell interactions, referred to commonly as the "seed and soil" hypothesis. He further went on to elaborate on this theory, stating "when a plant goes to seed, its seeds are carried in all directions, but they can only live and grow if they fall on congenial soil."

Even after more than 120 years, Paget's seed and soil hypothesis is the foundation of ongoing investigation. With continued refinement we may recognize the "seed" now as a progenitor cell, initiating cell, cancer stem cell, or metastatic cell, and the "soil" as a host factor, stroma, niche, or organ microenvironment.[23] In a more recent article on the biology of cancer metastasis, Talmadge and Fidler revised the concept of this hypothesis to include 3 main principles,[10] the first being that primary neoplasms (and metastases) consist of tumor and host cells. Host cells include epithelial cells, fibroblasts, endothelial cells, and infiltrating leukocytes. Furthermore, neoplasms contain biologically heterogeneous populations of tumor cells, each of which has the ability to complete some of the steps in metastatic process, but not all. The second principle is that the successful metastatic cells ("seed") are selected for their ability to succeed in invasion, embolization, survival in the circulation, arrest in a distant capillary bed, and extravasation into and multiplication within organ parenchyma. Metastasis favors the survival and growth of a few subpopulations of cells within the parent neoplasm, and current studies support a clonal origin for metastases. The third principle is that metastases develop in specific organs, or microenvironments ("soil"), which are biologically unique. There is a differential expression of cell-surface receptors and growth factors that can be either supportive of or inhospitable to metastases.[24,25]

THE BIOLOGY OF SUCCESSFUL METASTATIC CELLS ("SEED")

Successful metastatic cells are selected for their ability to undergo the processes of invasion, intravasation, arrest, extravasation, and colonization of distant organs.[10,26] Invasion initiates the metastatic process of a tumor cell, and involves changes in tumor cell adherence to other cells and to the extracellular matrix (ECM), disruption of the basement membrane and ECM, and motility to propel the tumor cell through tissue.

Loss of Adherence and Epithelial to Mesenchymal Transition

Integrins are mediators of tumor cell adherence to the ECM. Integrins exist as heterodimers that bind to specific proteins in the ECM and activate signaling pathways. In particular the $\alpha_6\beta_4$ integrin, which binds laminin on the ECM, signals through the oncogenic receptor tyrosine kinases Met, epithelial growth factor receptor, and Her2.[27] CD44 is also a tumor cell receptor for ECM-associated proteins. Integrins have also been implicated in later stages of metastasis: $\alpha_v\beta_3$ and $\alpha_3\beta_1$ integrins are involved in adhesions of circulating tumor cells to the vasculature,[28] and $\alpha_2\beta_1$ integrin has been demonstrated to bind to laminin-5 during lung metastasis.[29]

Cell-to-cell adhesion is regulated by cadherins,[4] which bind through protein-protein interactions on the extracellular domain and signal intracellularly to catenins and actin cytoskeleton.[30,31] Metastatic invasions is characterized by a change in cadherin expression consisting of a reduction in E-cadherin, which promotes tumor cell–tumor cell adherence, to an increase in N-cadherin, which is normally expressed on mesenchymal cells and facilitates tumor binding to the stroma during invasion.[26]

The loss of E-cadherin–associated adherence has been described in the larger context to resemble that of an epithelial to mesenchymal transition (EMT). EMT is vital process for morphogenesis during embryonic development, characterized by loss of epithelial cell polarity and cell-cell contacts. Concurrently, cells undergoing EMT acquire mesenchymal components and a migratory phenotype.[32] Given these phenotypic changes, EMT has gained interest among investigators in cancer metastasis as a mechanism to explain loss of epithelial adherence and gain of stromal mesenchymal invasion.

A significant feature of EMT is the loss of E-cadherin expression, which is consistently observed at sites of EMT during development and cancer. The loss of E-cadherin increases tumor invasiveness in vitro and contributes to a malignant phenotype in animal models.[32] Several genes have been identified that induce EMT and also act as E-cadherin repressors; these include Snail, Slug,[33] SIP1, and Twist.[34,35] The downregulation alone of E-cadherin is not sufficient for EMT,[32,34] and the loss of E-cadherin expression and cell adhesion do not define EMT. The acquisition of mesenchymal functions is also necessary for EMT. The prospective role of EMT in cancer metastasis and the continued elucidation of the numerous signaling pathways is a recently developing area of investigation, and may prove to offer an increased understanding of the process of metastasis and offer potential opportunities for therapeutic intervention.[36]

Cell Motility

A fundamental concept of metastasis is the transit of cells from one site to another. Most of this movement in tumor cells is a dynamic process involving the formation of adhesions to the ECM comprising cytoskeletal changes, proteolysis, and actin-myosin contractions.[5] Components of the cell motility machinery have been implicated in animal models of metastasis. The role of RhoC, a GTPase acting as a node of motility regulation, has been implicated in lung metastasis in an in vivo melanoma model.[36] Overexpression of Nedd9, a focal adhesion kinase adaptor protein, has been shown to foster cell motility and invasion in a mouse model of melanoma.[37] Furthermore, Nedd9 was identified as one of a set of genes that mediate lung metastasis in breast cancer.[38] Intravital imaging has demonstrated that tumor cells in vivo may move faster than once thought, based on in vitro experiments.[39] The purported increase in speed seems to be related to cells tracking along the collagenous ECM, and acquisition of this motility coincides with a metastatic phenotype.

Survival and Arrest in Transit

The ability to evade apoptosis is a significant feature of tumor cells; however, metastasizing tumor cells face a myriad of additional mechanical and physiologic barriers. Cell death can be triggered simply by velocity-induced shear forces of the bloodstream or by hypoxia and nutrient deprivation. The loss of extracellular attachment can induce cell death, so-called death by detachment or anoikis. Loss of expression of caspase-8, an apoptotic initiator caspase, facilitates metastasis by increasing the resistance of a tumor cell to anoikis.[40] The brain-derived neurotrophic factor receptor trkB was shown in vitro to confer resistance to anoikis in tumor cells, and contributed to a metastatic phenotype.[41] Furthermore, overexpression of antiapoptotic effector genes such as BCL2, BCL-X, and XIAP in tumor cells can make them more resilient to death stimuli.[42]

Metastasizing cancer cells must not only survive in circulation but also eventually arrest in capillary beds. Circulating tumor cells may shield themselves with platelets, creating a tumor embolus that is purported to be more resistant to immune-mediated clearance and shear hemodynamic stress.[43] Mechanical lodging of platelet-tumor emboli is likely a prevalent form of tumor arrest in capillary beds of distant organs. Other proposed mechanisms of arrest involve receptor–cognate ligand interactions. The $\alpha_2\beta_1$ integrin expressed on a cancer cell has been demonstrated to bind to laminin-5 within exposed regions of the vascular basement membrane during lung metastasis.[29] Tumor cells have also been demonstrated to bind other coagulation factors including tissue factor, fibrin, fibrinogen, and thrombin to create a tumor embolus that aids in capillary arrest.[26]

Extravasation

The metastasizing tumor cell that survives the circulation and arrests in a distant organ capillary bed must now transit from the vascular endothelium into a target organ in a process referred to as extravasation. Methods of extravasation differ in various tumor types. The process can occur by sheer mechanical stress as the tumor grows to substantial size and erupts into the adjacent tissue vasculature.[44] In osteosarcoma, ezrin, a cytoskeletal protein, has been demonstrated to contribute to metastatic extravasation into lung tissue.[45] More recently, the vascular endothelial growth factor receptor (VEGFR) has been identified as a potential mediator of extravasation by disrupting endothelial cell junctions in target tissue vasculature through activation of Src family kinases.[46] Animal models have shown that VEGF-secreting tumor cells were unable to metastasize to lungs of Src knockout mice.[47]

THE BIOLOGY OF THE ORGAN MICROENVIRONMENT ("SOIL")

Successful colonization of the distant organ by the metastatic cancer cell ("seed") depends on the interaction with the microenvironment of the tissue ("soil"). Clinical observations have revealed distinct that tumor phenotypes metastasize to specific organs, independent of the volume of exposure or blood supply. The use of peritoneovenous shunts to palliate ascites for women with advanced ovarian cancer has demonstrated that the high volume exposure of cancer cells to an organ via the circulatory system is inadequate alone to form metastatic disease. Tarin and colleagues[48] described that despite dissemination of millions of cancer cells into the circulation, metastatic disease in the lungs, the first organ capillary bed, was rare.

The definition of a microenvironment continues to evolve concurrent with our increasing understanding of the processes that govern it. At present, the microenvironment appears to include a cellular architecture and a "premetastatic niche" created by the influx of supporting cells to support the process of metastasis.[49] Kaplan and colleagues[49] have demonstrated that VEGFR1-positive hematopoietic bone marrow progenitor cells target tumor-specific premetastatic sites and form cellular clusters that are conducive to the formation of metastatic disease. These cells further create a permissive niche for metastasis by expressing integrin $\alpha_4\beta_1$ and upregulating fibronectin in resident fibroblasts.

Pulmonary metastasis is a relatively common pattern of metastatic disease that can be seen among an array of primary tumors, including breast cancer, gastrointestinal tumors, melanoma, sarcoma, and renal cancer. The ability of organ-specific colonization depends on a favorable microenvironment and characteristics of the tumor cells that interact favorably in this niche. A contributing factor may be the exposure of the capillary bed of the lungs to the entire circulatory volume. Furthermore, specific genes have been implicated in pulmonary metastasis. The cytoskeletal anchoring protein, ezrin, seems to contribute to tumor cell extravasation into lung parenchyma, and its expression correlates negatively in osteosarcoma patients.[45] In breast cancer, the pathways of nuclear factor κB and transforming growth factor β have been associated with lung metastasis.[50,51]

SUMMARY

The process of metastasis relies on a series of stochastic and sequential steps, with selective pressure exerted on a large number of genetically volatile cancer cells to produce a very small fraction of tumor cells with the ability to navigate the transition from primary tumor cell to end-organ metastasis. This process is intricately determined by cell-microenvironment interactions, the mechanistic understanding of which is steadily increasing. The continued elucidation of pathways that govern these interactions offers potential therapeutic options to patients with advanced disease.

REFERENCES

1. Paget S. The distribution of secondary growths in cancer of the breast. Lancet 1889;133:571–3.
2. Fidler IJ, Gersten DM, Kripke ML. Influence of immune status on the metastasis of three murine

fibrosarcomas of different immunogenicities. Cancer Res 1979;39:3816–21.

3. Weidner N, Semple JP, Welch WR, et al. Tumor angiogenesis and metastasis-correlation in invasive breast carcinoma. N Engl J Med 1991;324:1–8.

4. Cavallaro U, Christofori G. Cell adhesion and signaling by cadherins and IG-CAMs in cancer. Nat Rev Cancer 2004;4:118–32.

5. Friedl P, Wolf K. Tumour-cell invasion and migration: diversity and escape mechanisms. Nat Rev Cancer 2003;3:362–74.

6. Egeblad M, Werb Z. New functions for the matrix metalloproteinases in cancer progression. Nat Rev Cancer 2002;2:161–74.

7. Liotta LA, Kohn EC. The microenvironment of the tumor-host interface. Nature 2001;411:375–9.

8. Sugarbaker EV. Cancer metastasis: a product of tumor-host interactions. Curr Probl Cancer 1979;0: 1–59.

9. Nicolson GL, Brunson KW, Fidler IJ. Specificity of arrest, survival, and growth of selected metastatic variant cell lines. Cancer Res 1978;38:4105–11.

10. Talmadge JE, Fidler IJ. AACR centennial series: the biology of cancer metastasis: historical perspective. Cancer Res 2010;70:5649–69.

11. Chambers AF, Groom AC, MacDonald IC. Dissemination and growth of cancer cells in metastatic sites. Nat Rev Cancer 2002;2:563–72.

12. Fidler IJ, Kripke ML. Metastasis results from preexisting variant cells within a malignant tumor. Science 1977;197:893–5.

13. Fidler IJ, Gruys E, Cifone MA, et al. Demonstration of multiple phenotypic diversity in a murine melanoma of recent origin. J Natl Cancer Inst 1981;67: 947–56.

14. Gupta GP, Massague J. Cancer metastasis: building a framework. Cell 2006;127:679–95.

15. Hernando E, Nahle Z, Juan G, et al. Rb inactivation promotes genomic instability by uncoupling cell cycle progression from mitotic control. Nature 2004; 430:797–802.

16. Puc J, Keniry M, Li HS, et al. Lack of PTEN sequesters CHK1 and initiates genetic instability. Cancer Cell 2005;7:193–204.

17. Maser RS, DePinho RA. Connecting chromosomes, crisis and cancer. Science 2002;297:565–9.

18. Baylin SB, Ohm JE. Epigenetic gene silencing in cancer—a mechanism for early oncogenic pathway addiction? Nat Rev Cancer 2006;6:107–16.

19. Feinberg AP, Ohlsson R, Henrikoff S. The epigenetic progenitor origin of human cancer. Nat Rev Genet 2006;7:21–33.

20. Nowell PC. The clonal evolution of tumor cell populations. Science 1976;194:23–8.

21. Talmadge JE, Wolman SR, Fidler IJ. Evidence for the clonal origin of spontaneous metastases. Science 1982;217:361–3.

22. Jones TD, Carr MD, Eble JN. Clonal origin of lymph node metastases in bladder carcinoma. Cancer 2005;104:1901–10.

23. Langley RR, Fidler IJ. Tumor cell-organ microenvironment interactions in the pathogenesis of cancer metastasis. Endocr Rev 2007;28:297–321.

24. Pasqualini R, Ruoslahti E. Organ targeting in vivo using phage display peptide libraries. Nature 1996; 380:364–6.

25. Uehara H, Kim SJ, Karashima T, et al. Effects of blocking platelet-derived growth factor-receptor signaling in a mouse model of experimental prostate cancer bone metastases. J Natl Cancer Inst 2003; 95:458–70.

26. Steeg PS. Tumor metastasis: mechanistic insights and clinical challenges. Nat Med 2006;12:895–904.

27. Guo W, Giancotti FG. Integrin signaling during tumour progression. Nat Rev Mol Cell Biol 2004;5: 816–26.

28. Felding-Habermann B, O'Toole TE, Smith JW, et al. Integrin activation controls metastasis in human breast cancer. Proc Natl Acad Sci U S A 2001;98: 1853–8.

29. Wang H, Fu W, Im JH, et al. Tumor cell alpha3beta1 integrin and vascular laminin-5 mediate pulmonary arrest and metastasis. J Cell Biol 2004;164:935–41.

30. Beavon IG. The E-cadherin-catenin complex in tumour metastasis: structure, function and regulation. Eur J Cancer 2000;36:1607–20.

31. Bremnes RM, Veve R, Hirsch FR, et al. The E-cadherin cell-cell adhesion complex and lung cancer invasion, metastasis, and prognosis. Lung Cancer 2002;36:115–24.

32. Thiery JP. Epithelial-mesenchymal transitions in tumour progression. Nat Rev Cancer 2002;6:442–54.

33. Nieto MA. The snail superfamily of zinc-finger transcription factors. Nat Rev Mol Cell Biol 2002;3: 155–66.

34. Yang J, Mani SA, Donaher JL, et al. Twist, a master regulator of morphogenesis, plays an essential role in tumor metastasis. Cell 2004;117:927–39.

35. Talbot LJ, Bhattacharya SD, Kuo PC. Epithelial-mesenchymal transition, the tumor microenvironment, and metastatic behavior of epithelial malignancies. Int J Biochem Mol Biol 2012;2:117–36.

36. Clark EA, Golub TR, Lander ES, et al. Genomic analysis of metastasis reveals an essential role for RhoC. Nature 2000;406:532–5.

37. Kim M, Gans JD, Nogueira C, et al. Comparative oncogenomics identifies NEDD9 as a melanoma metastasis gene. Cell 2006;125:1269–81.

38. Minn AJ, Gupta GP, Siegel PM, et al. Genes that mediate breast cancer metastasis to lung. Nature 2005;436:518–24.

39. Condeelis J, Segall JE. Intravital imaging of cell movement in tumours. Nat Rev Cancer 2003;3: 921–30.

40. Stupack DG, Teitz T, Potter MD, et al. Potentiation of neuroblastoma metastasis by loss of caspase-8. Nature 2006;439:95–9.

41. Douma S, Van Laar T, Zevenhoven J, et al. Suppression of anoikis and induction of metastasis by the neurotrophic receptor TrkB. Nature 2004;430:1034–9.

42. Mehlen P, Puisieux A. Metastasis: a question of life or death. Nat Rev Cancer 2006;6:449–58.

43. Nash GF, Turner LF, Scully MF, et al. Platelets and cancer. Lancet Oncol 2002;3:425–30.

44. Al-Mehdi AB, Tozawa K, Fisher AB, et al. Intravascular origin of metastasis from the proliferation of endothelium-attached tumor cells: a new model for metastasis. Nat Med 2000;6:100–2.

45. Khanna C, Wan X, Bose S, et al. The membrane-cytoskeleton liner ezrin is necessary for osteosarcoma metastasis. Nat Med 2004;10:182–6.

46. Weis SM, Cheresh DA. Pathophysiological consequences of VEGF-induced vascular permeability. Nature 2005;437:497–504.

47. Criscuoli ML, Nguyen M, Eliceiri BP. Tumor metastasis but not tumor growth is dependent on Src-mediated vascular permeability. Blood 2005;105:1508–14.

48. Tarin D, Price JE, Kettlewell MG, et al. Mechanisms of human tumor metastasis studied in patients with peritoneovenous shunts. Cancer Res 1984;44:3584–92.

49. Kaplan RN, Riba RD, Zacharoulis S, et al. VEGFR1-positive haematopoietic bone marrow progenitors initiate the pre-metastatic niche. Nature 2005;438:820–7.

50. Luo JL, Maeda S, Hsu LC, et al. Inhibition of NF-kappaB in cancer cells converts inflammation-induced tumor growth mediated by TNFalpha to TRAIL-mediated tumor regression. Cancer Cell 2004;6:297–305.

51. Siegel PM, Shu W, Cardiff RD, et al. Transforming growth factor beta signaling impairs Neu-induced mammary tumorigenesis while promoting pulmonary metastasis. Proc Natl Acad Sci U S A 2003;100:8430–5.

Preoperative Evaluation and Indications for Pulmonary Metastasectomy

Loretta Erhunmwunsee, MD[a], Betty C. Tong, MD, MHS[b],*

KEYWORDS

- Pulmonary • Metastasectomy • Indications • Evaluation

KEY POINTS

- Only 15% to 25% of patients with pulmonary metastases will be appropriate candidates for surgery.
- Preoperative evaluation of pulmonary metastasectomy patients has 2 goals: first, to determine a patient's fitness for surgery; and second, to determine whether the pulmonary metastases are resectable.
- Individuals should undergo pulmonary metastasectomy under the following conditions: 1. the primary tumor site is controlled; 2. there is no evidence of extrathoracic metastases or these metastases are controlled; 3. the pulmonary metastases are completely resectable and resection will leave adequate pulmonary function; 4. there is no medical management with lower morbidity that can be offered in lieu of surgery.

PREOPERATIVE EVALUATION

The purpose of preoperative evaluation of patients referred for pulmonary metastasectomy is twofold.[1-3] The first component focuses on defining the morbidity, risks of surgery, and specific factors in patients that can be addressed to decrease the patient's operative risk. Secondly, the evaluation determines whether the lesions are actually resectable. In assessing the patient's fitness for surgery, it is important to remember that the most common complications after major thoracic surgery include pneumonia, atelectasis, atrial fibrillation, and heart failure.[4] Most patients who undergo pulmonary metastasectomy undergo thoracoscopic wedge resection, but larger resections and the need for thoracotomy are possible. Therefore, it is key to assess the cardiac and pulmonary reserve of a patient being

evaluated for pulmonary metastasectomy, especially if a larger or more complex resection is potentially required.

History and Physical Examination

Every preoperative evaluation should begin with a history and physical examination. Although up to 90% of patients with pulmonary metastases will be asymptomatic secondary to the nonobstructing peripheral nature of their disease, the history should start with an assessment of respiratory symptoms. If the patient has respiratory symptoms, then the individual may have endobronchial or pleural involvement, large bulky disease, or a central tumor.[5] Next, the history should determine a patient's functional status. Asking the patient and family about his or her actual daily activities can be enlightening. If it is apparent that the

Disclosures: The authors have nothing to disclose.
[a] Division of Thoracic Surgery, City of Hope Comprehensive Cancer Center, 1500 East Duarte Road, Duarte, CA 91010, USA; [b] Division of Cardiovascular and Thoracic Surgery, Department of Surgery, Duke University Medical Center, DUMC Box 3531, Durham, NC 27710, USA
* Corresponding author.
E-mail address: betty.tong@duke.edu

Thorac Surg Clin 26 (2016) 7–12
http://dx.doi.org/10.1016/j.thorsurg.2015.09.002
1547-4127/16/$ – see front matter © 2016 Elsevier Inc. All rights reserved.

patient's activity level is quite low, then further evaluation of his or her fitness for surgery should occur; objective assessments such as a 6-minute walk test or cardiopulmonary exercise testing are often revealing.

During the history, the patient must also be evaluated for symptoms of metastases to other locations (eg, recent fractures, bone pain, new headaches, or other neurologic events or symptoms). A history of pulmonary and cardiac diseases and other comorbidites such as diabetes or renal or liver disease must also be elicted. Medications should be discussed and a perioperative plan made for anticoagulants, immunosuppression, and cardiac medications. Also, social history should be evaluated and screening for substance abuse completed. Current smokers should be required, or at least strongly encouraged, to stop smoking prior to surgery, and they should be provided with smoking cessation resources and education. Alcohol users should also be asked about use, in order to prevent and treat potential withdrawal symptoms. Although it may not be particularly revealing, a physical examination should be performed. A patient with wheezing on examination may have endobronchial disease, or an individual with a pericardial rub have pericardial involvement, for example.

Imaging

Evaluation of the pulmonary lesions typically begins with a chest computed tomography (CT) scan, which has a high detection rate of metastatic pulmonary nodules.[6] McCormack and colleagues[7] have found that despite the use of these high-resolution, thin-section chest CTs that 20% to 25% of nodules are still not imaged, suggesting that operative manual palpation must be performed. As CT scanning technology evolves, the detection of nodules as small as 1 mm is being achieved, further narrowing the disparity between CT scanning and manual palpation.[6]

Positron emission tomography (PET) scans are frequently performed on patients with epithelial-based primary tumors and melanoma after an abnormality on a CT scan is discovered. The use of these scans in the preoperative evaluation of lung lesions continues to rise. Mayerhoefer and colleagues[8] analyzed the utility of PET in a study of 181 patients with pulmonary metastases. The PET sensitivity was 7.9% for lesions of 4 to 5 mm, 33.3% for lesions 6 to 7 mm, 56.8% for lesions 8 to 9 mm, 63.6% for lesions 10 to 11 mm, and lesions 100% for 12 mm or higher ($P<.0010$); thus the larger the lesion, the more sensitive the PET results.

Bamba and colleagues[9] found that pulmonary metastasis of colorectal cancer can be accurately diagnosed by PET/CT, especially when nodules are larger than 9 mm in greatest dimension. Xi and colleagues[10] performed a meta-analysis and found that fluorodeoxyglucos (FDG) PET/CT was a valuable diagnostic tool for diagnosing lung malignancies in patients with head and neck squamous cell cancer, with a sensitivity of 85% and specificity of 98%. In a series by Fortes and colleagues,[11,12] the sensitivity of PET was evaluated in a series of 83 patients who underwent a pulmonary metastasectomy. In this series, the PET scan was positive in only 67.5% of the malignant nodules (colon, 68.6%; renal cell carcinoma, 71.4%; sarcoma, 44.4%), revealing that PET has its shortcomings. Franzius and colleagues[13] suggest that there is a superiority of spiral CT in the detection of pulmonary metastases from malignant primary bone tumors as compared with FDG-PET. They found spiral CT to have higher sensitivity, specificity, and accuracy than FDG-PET in detecting pulmonary metastases from malignant primary bone tumors.[14,15] Thus chest, abdomen, and pelvic CT scans are frequently the only imaging used in evaluating patients with a history of sarcoma; however, it is not unreasonable to use PET also.

Mediastinal Staging

Mediastinal and hilar lymph nodes should also be evaluated on the preoperative imaging. Lymph node involvement is an important negative prognostic factor in patients undergoing metastasectomy regardless of histology.[16–18] For that reason, those with mediastinal adenopathy may benefit from surgical staging by mediastinoscopy or endobronchial ultrasound (EBUS) fine needle aspiration (FNA) before pulmonary metastasectomy is performed. Although patients with hilar or mediastinal lymph node involvement have poorer survival than those without, the presence of documented nodal metastasis is not an absolute contraindication for metastasectomy as there are some patients with lymph node involvement who are long-term survivors after metastasectomy.[17]

Pulmonary Function Testing

Pulmonary function testing is an important component to the preoperative evaluation of those who are undergoing an anatomic resection of metastatic lesions. The postoperative diffusion capacity (DLCO) and forced expiratory volume at 1 second (FEV_1) must be determined, as they are important predictors of operative risk, postoperative complications, and even mortality. Although sub-lobar resection (either wedge resection or seg-mentectomy) is most often used for patients undergoing metastasectomy, one must consider the potential cumulative parenchymal loss in the setting of multiple lesions. In one study, patients who had at least 3 nonanatomic resections had pulmonary functional losses similar to those un-dergoing lobectomy.[19] Given this, it is not unrea-sonable to apply similar standards for baseline pulmonary function for patients in need of meta-stasectomy as for lung cancer resection. Current guidelines suggest that patients with a predicted postoperative FEV_1 or DLCO between 30% and 60% predicted should have additional risk stratifi-cation with an exercise test, such as a shuttle walk test or stair climb, prior to proceeding with sur-gery. Patients with postoperative predicted FEV_1 or DLCO less than 30% should undergo formal cardiopulmonary exercise testing with measure-ment of maximal oxygen consumption.[20]

Evaluation of Extrathoracic Metastasis

It is estimated that 75% or more of patients with pulmonary nodules will also have metastases to extrathoracic sites. Only 15% to 25% of patients have lesions confined to the lung and are appro-priate candidates for curative resection.[5] For this reason, staging for metastatic disease outside of the lung is performed prior to pulmonary resection, based on the primary tumor. In most patients, CT of the chest and abdomen is performed to exclude liver metastases. For patients with sarcoma, PET scan or bone scan may be performed to assess for the presence of bone metastases.[21] PET scan is also commonly used to assess metastatic disease in patients with epithelial tumors and melanoma. Any patient with pulmonary metasta-ses who presents with neurologic symptoms should undergo brain imaging with either MRI or CT scan with and without contrast to exclude involvement of the central nervous system. Some clinicians routinely obtain brain imaging in patients with metastatic melanoma, breast cancer, or colon cancer, as each frequently metastasizes to the brain.[22]

Summary

Preoperative evaluation for patients undergoing pulmonary metastasectomy determines whether the patient is fit for surgery. A focused history and physical examination are the cornerstones of this component of the evaluation, and the use of cardiopulmonary testing can be vital for those with low activity or poor pulmonary function. The preoperative evaluation also determines whether the lesions are completely resectable. One should seriously consider the risks and benefits to debulk-ing if the lesions are not completely resectable. CT and PET assess the parenchymal, lymph node, and extrathoracic involvement. Surgical staging may also be required before metastasectomy if there is suspicion of mediastinal adenopathy on imaging. If anatomic resections are planned, then evaluation must include pulmonary function testing also.

INDICATIONS FOR METASTASECTOMY

The purpose of pulmonary metastasectomy is predominantly for curative intent, but a diag-nostic wedge may be performed simply for tis-sue diagnosis or for evaluation of residual disease after other therapy as well.[5] Here the focus is on describing the indications of pulmo-nary metastasectomy performed for curative intent.

The criteria for pulmonary metastasectomy were originally described 6 decades ago:

1. Candidates should be of appropriate risk for surgical intervention.
2. The primary malignancy must to be controllable
3. There should not be evidence of metastatic dis-ease in any other part of the body.
4. Imaging should show only metastases to one lung.[23–27]

The criteria adopted today are still similar to those of Ehrenhaft and Thomford; although with anesthetic, surgical, radiologic and critical care advances, some of the criteria have been expanded. Today the criteria include

1. The primary malignancy must be controlled or controllable.
2. There is no extrathoracic metastasis that is not controlled or controllable.
3. All of the tumor must be resectable, with adequate remaining pulmonary reserve.
4. There are no alternative medical treatment options with lower morbidity.

Each of these criteria must be met before offer-ing surgery and will be discussed separately.

Primary Malignancy Must be Controlled or Controllable

When a patient is found to have pulmonary metas-tases, it is imperative that his or her site of primary malignancy is thoroughly evaluated. Patients will not obtain a survival benefit from metastesectomy if their primary tumor is not controlled. Whether the metastasis is discovered metachronously or synchronously, the primary site must be investigated to determine whether the tumor or local recurrence is controllable. If the primary site is still present when metastases are discovered, resection of the primary should be achieved prior to metastasectomy. However, in this situation, a trial of systemic therapy followed by reassessment of the disease burden, rather than serial resection of the primary site and metastatic disease, should be strongly considered. Patients with colon cancer will need to undergo colonoscopy and abdominal/pelvic CT once a metastasis is noted. Patients with current or a history of breast cancer should undergo mammography. Head and neck cancer patients benefit from examination under anesthesia with endoscopy and contrasted neck CT, while those with a history of renal cancer frequently undergo a contrasted abdominal CT scan or MRI for better evaluation of the primary tumor. Melanoma patients should have a full skin evaluation by a dermatologist, and sarcoma patients should have CT, MRI, and/or bone scan performed to evaluate their site of primary malignancy. Patients with germ cell tumors should undergo blood work analysis of β-HCG, α-fetoprotein, and lactate dehydrogenase (LDH) as well as evaluation of the testes with ultrasound as necessary. If evaluation determines that a primary tumor is unresectable, then pulmonary metastesectomy should generally not be pursued.

Extrathoracic Metastasis Must be Controlled or Controllable

In almost all cases, extrathoracic metastases are a contraindication for pulmonary metastasectomy performed for curative intent; therefore the presence of metastatic disease outside the lungs excludes the patient from surgery. The exception to this rule is for patients with limited, resectable hepatic metastases from colon cancer in the setting of pulmonary metastases. There has been no reported difference in outcome in patients with and without history of previously resected hepatic metastases at the time of pulmonary resection, and thus many perform pulmonary metastasectomy even in patients who have undergone hepatic resection for colorectal metastases at an earlier stage.[18,28] Patients who undergo combination hepatic and pulmonary metastasectomy have a 30% 5-year survival rate.[28] Pfannschmidt and colleagues[18] found similar results with no significant difference in outcome observed between patients with and without history of previously resected hepatic metastases at the time of pulmonary resection, with 5-year survival rates between 30% and 42%.

As a rule, patients with extrathoracic metastases other than limited hepatic tumors should not undergo pulmonary metastasectomy for curative intent. Those who are being considered for such should be evaluated in a multidisciplinary tumor board.

All of the Tumor Must be Completely Resectable with Adequate Remaining Pulmonary Reserve

An appraisal of the ability to achieve complete resection with adequate pulmonary reserve is vital and includes evaluation of the number of nodules, consideration of the location of nodules, and estimation of the postoperative pulmonary function. Data from the International Registry of Lung Metastases indicate better 5-year survival rates for patients with a single metastatic focus (43% 5 year survival) when compared with those with 2 to 3 metastases (34%) or those with 3 or more metastases (27%).[24] For patients with multiple metastases, there is no consensus as to how many lesions is too many. At this time, if lesions can be completely cleared while allowing for adequate remaining function, then resection can be pursued even if the lesions are numerous, bilateral or if anatomic resection such as segmentectomy or lobectomy is required. In the case of potential pneumonectomy, a thorough discussion of alternative therapies, in a multidisciplinary setting, should be conducted prior to embarking upon surgery.

No Superior Alternative Nonoperative Management

For most tumor histologies, there is no medical option that has a proven survival advantage over pulmonary metastasectomy. The exceptions are patients with nonseminomatous germ cell tumors and potentially those with breast cancer. When patients present with lung metastases from these etiologies, discussion with the medical oncologist should occur, as there are chemotherapeutic and hormonal therapies that can be offered for curative intent, without the risks of surgery.

SUMMARY

Most patients with pulmonary metastases will not be candidates for pulmonary metastasectomy. Preoperative evaluation determines whether a patient is both fit enough for surgery and has disease that is actually resectable and potentially curable. Both components are necessary in patients who undergo resection for curative intent. In general, to be considered for pulmonary metastasectomy, patients must fit several criteria:

- The primary disease is controlled.
- Any extrathoracic disease is controlled.
- Complete resection of pulmonary involvement is achievable with adequate pulmonary reserve.
- There are no effective medical therapies.

REFERENCES

1. Welter S, Jacobs J, Krbek T, et al. Pulmonary metastases of breast cancer. When is resection indicated? Eur J Cardiothorac Surg 2008;34: 1228–34.
2. Erhunmwunsee L, D'Amico TA. Surgical management of pulmonary metastases. Ann Thorac Surg 2009;88:2052–60.
3. Kaifi JT, Gusani NJ, Deshaies I, et al. Indications and approach to surgical resection of lung metastases. J Surg Oncol 2010;102:187–95.
4. Reilly JJ. Preoperative Evaluation of Patients Undergoing Thoracic Surgery. In: Selke FW, del Nido PJ, Swanson SJ, editors. Sabiston and Spencer Surgery of the Chest. Philadelphia: Saunders Elsevier; 2010. p. 39–46.
5. Cowan S, Culligan M, Friedberg J. Secondary Lung Tumors. In: Selke FW, del Nido PJ, Swanson SJ, editors. Sabiston and Spencer Surgery of the Chest. Philadelphia: Saunders Elsevier; 2010. p. 337–50.
6. Kang MC, Kang CH, Lee HJ, et al. Accuracy of 16-channel multi-detector row chest computed tomography with thin sections in the detection of metastatic pulmonary nodules. Eur J Cardiothorac Surg 2008;33:473–9.
7. McCormack PM, Ginsberg KB, Bains MS, et al. Accuracy of lung imaging in metastases with implications for the role of thoracoscopy. Ann Thorac Surg 1993;56(4):863–5; discussion 865–6.
8. Mayerhoefer ME, Prosch H, Herold CJ, et al. Assessment of pulmonary melanoma metastases with 18F-FDG PET/CT: Which PET-negative patients require additional tests for definitive staging? Eur Radiol 2012;22(11):2451–7.
9. Bamba Y, Itabashi M, Kameoka S. Value of PET/CT imaging for diagnosing pulmonary metastasis of colorectal cancer. Hepatogastroenterology 2011; 58:1972–4.
10. Xi K, Xie X, Xi S. Meta-analysis of 18 fluorodeoxyglucose positron emission tomography–CT for diagnosis of lung malignancies in patients with head and neck squamous cell carcinomas. Head Neck 2015;37(11):1680–4.
11. Fortes DL, Allen MS, Lowe VJ, et al. The sensitivity of 18F-flourodeoxyglucose positron emission tomography in the evaluation of metastatic pulmonary nodules. Eur J Cardiothorac Surg 2008;34: 1223–7.
12. Mayerhoefer ME, Prosch H, Herold CJ, et al. Assessment of pulmonary melanoma metastases with 18 F-FDG PET/CT: which PET-negative patients require additional tests for definitive staging? Eur Radiology 2012;22:2451–7.
13. Franzius C, Daldrup-Link HE, Sciuk J, et al. FDG-PET for detection of pulmonary metastases from malignant primary bone tumors: comparison with spiral CT. Ann Oncol 2001;12(4):479–86.
14. Metser U, You J, McSweeney S, et al. Assessment of tumor recurrence in patients with colorectal cancer and elevated carcinoembryonic antigen level: FDG PET/CT versus contrast-enhanced 64-MDCT of the chest and abdomen. AJR Am J Roentgenol 2010; 194(3):766–71.
15. Higashiyama M, Tokunaga T, Nakagiri T, et al. Pulmonary metastasetomy: outcomes and issues according to the type of surgical resection. Gen Thorac Cardiovasc Surg 2015;63(6):320–30.
16. Hamaji M, Cassivi SD, Shen KR, et al. Is lymph node dissection required in pulmonary metastasectomy for colorectal adenocarcinoma? Ann Thorac Surg 2012;94:1796–800.
17. Murthy SC, Kim K, Rice TW, et al. Can we predict long-term survival after pulmonary metastasectomy for renal cell carcinoma? Ann Thorac Surg 2005; 79:996–1003.
18. Pfannschmidt J, Dienemann H, Hoffmann J. Surgical resection of pulmonary metastases from colorectal cancer: a systematic review of published series. Ann Thorac Surg 2007;84:324–38.
19. Petrella F, Chieco P, Solli P, et al. Which factors affect pulmonary function after lung metastasectomy? Eur J Cardiothorac Surg 2009;35(5):792–6.
20. Brunelli A, Kim AW, Berger KI, et al. Physiologic evaluation of the patient with lung cancer being considered for resectional surgery. Chest 2013; 143(5 Suppl):e166S–90S.
21. National Comprehensive Cancer Network: clinical practice guidelines in oncology: soft tissue sarcoma. Available at: http://www.nccn.org/professionals/physician_gls/f_guidelines.asp. Accessed April 19, 2015.
22. Jaklitsch MT, Burt BM, Jett JR, et al. Surgical resection of pulmonary metastases: Benefits, indications, preoperative evaluation and techniques. In: Friedberg JS, editor. UpToDate. Waltham (MA): UpToDate; 2015.
23. Kondo H, Okumura T, Ohde Y, et al. Surgical treatment for metastatic malignancies. Pulmonary metastasisi: indications and outcomes. Int J Clin Oncol 2005;10:81–5.
24. Pastorino U, Buyse M, Friedel G, et al. Long-term results of lung metastasectomy: prognostic analyses

based on 5206 cases. J Thorac Cardiovasc Surg 1997;113:37–49.

25. Mountain CF, McMurtrey MJ, Hermes KE. Surgery for pulmonary metastasis: a 20-year experience. J Thorac Cardiovasc Surg 1984;38:323–9.

26. Ehrenhaft JL, Lawrence MS, Sensenig DM. Pulmonary resection for metastatic lesions. Arch Surg 1958;77:606–12.

27. Thomford NR, Woolner LB, Clagett OT, et al. The surgical treatment of metastatic tumors in the lungs. J Thorac Cardiovasc Surg 1965;49: 357–63.

28. Joosten J, Betholet J, Keemers-Gels M, et al. Pulmonary resetion of colorectal metastases in patients with or without a history of hepatic metastases. Eur J Surg Oncol 2008;34:895–9.

Open Surgical Approaches for Pulmonary Metastasectomy

Robert J. Downey, MD*, Manjit S. Bains, MD

KEYWORDS

- Pulmonary metastasectomy • Surgical approaches • Thoracotomy • Open approaches

KEY POINTS

- Both video-assisted thoracic surgical techniques and open thoracotomy are accepted as appropriate incisions for performing pulmonary metastasectomy.
- Open techniques have been shown to lead to the detection and hence, resection of more metastases than VATS techniques.
- Retrospective studies suggest that this improved detection and resection with open techniques does not lead to improved survival after surgery.
- The technical aspects of the various thoracotomy techniques are reviewed.

BACKGROUND

Resection of pulmonary metastases from nonpulmonary primary malignancies has been widely adopted with the goal of cure. Thoughtful surgeons differ in the approach to such resections, with some favoring procedures that minimize the trauma to the patient, and others performing open procedures with the goal of maximizing the likelihood of resection of all detectable sites of disease. In this article, we review how pulmonary metastasectomy emerged as a therapy for metastatic disease, focusing on how surgical approaches used for this procedure have evolved; the available literature addressing whether open procedures lead to more complete resections; and if so, whether resection by open procedures increases the likelihood of cure following resection. After this background, we review the technical aspects of the various thoracotomy techniques.

The first English language report was by Edwards[1] in 1927 of a subtotal lobectomy for pulmonary recurrence 6 years after lower extremity amputation for a sarcoma. The criteria for suitability were established first by Alexander and Haight in 1947[2] and remain by and large appropriate today. They are (1) the primary site of disease is controlled or controllable, (2) there should be no evidence for extrapulmonary metastatic disease, and (3) the patient must be able to tolerate the resection. In addition, as newer effective therapies have emerged, there should be no better alternative therapy (eg, the highly effective use of chemotherapy for germ cell tumors has reduced the need for pulmonary resection). The first pulmonary metastasectomy was performed at Memorial Hospital in 1940, and in line with the general practice adopted by the thoracic surgical community, subsequently was offered primarily to patients with one or two metastases and with long disease-free intervals (DFIs) (**Fig. 1**).

Over the years, there have been many hundreds of publications on the subject of pulmonary metastasectomy. By and large, these studies suffer from multiple deficiencies. For example, they combine diverse histologies that likely should be treated as separate diseases; and patients in a given study are often treated with varying induction and adjuvant chemotherapy and radiation

Thoracic Service, Department of Surgery, Memorial Hospital, Memorial Sloan-Kettering Cancer Center, 1275 York Avenue, New York, NY 10065, USA
* Corresponding author.
E-mail address: downeyr@mskcc.org

Thorac Surg Clin 26 (2016) 13–18
http://dx.doi.org/10.1016/j.thorsurg.2015.09.003

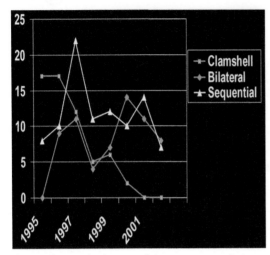

Fig. 1. Changes in the use of thoracotomy techniques at Memorial Hospital for resection of bilateral pulmonary metastases.

therapy regimens, which clouds the added benefit of surgical resection. Most importantly, all of the published series are retrospective and therefore that denominator of all patients with the disease from which the surgical patients are selected is not known. A fair criticism of these studies is that patients selected for surgery may represent those with indolent disease who may have experienced prolonged survival without resection.

Some retrospective evidence for efficacy is compelling. For example, members of the orthopedic service at Memorial Hospital noted that of 145 pediatric patients who underwent resection of extremity osteogenic sarcomas, 83% developed pulmonary metastases within 2 years, all of whom died within next 2 years.[3] Subsequently, Martini and colleagues[4] resected metastases from 22 patients who experienced a 32% 5-year and an 18% 20-year survival. The strongest evidence for the probable benefit from metastasectomy was developed by Pastorino and colleagues[5] who developed a registry of 5206 patients from 18 international centers and identified risk stratification factors including completeness of resection, a DFI of 36 months, and one versus more than one metastasis. Patients with one metastasis and a DFI of more than 3 years were found to have a 5-year survival of approximately 60%, whereas patients with more than one metastasis and a DFI of less than 3 months had a 5-year survival of approximately 30%. Currently, the PulMICC trial (A Randomized Trial of Pulmonary Metastasectomy in Colorectal Cancer), a phase III trial[6] randomizing patients to resection or best medical therapy, is accruing well and it is hoped will provide stronger evidence of which patients are likely to benefit from metastasectomy.

INTRODUCTION OF VIDEO-ASSISTED THORACIC SURGERY TECHNIQUES

Beginning about 1995, minimally invasive surgical techniques (video-assisted thoracic surgery [VATS]) were introduced into thoracic surgical practice and applied to pulmonary metastasectomy (**Fig. 2**). VATS techniques were assessed for oncologic safety[7] and it is likely that as techniques have matured, VATS procedures are no more or less likely than open techniques to disseminate disease. Concerns were also raised that VATS might be less effective than open procedures at achieving the first of the Alexander and Haight criteria discussed previously, that is, that the metastases be completely resected. Open thoracotomy incisions allow palpation of at least one lung, and it was noted that routinely nonradiographically evident metastases would be found by palpation. Because resection of all disease was believed to be important and because a posterolateral thoracotomy allowed evaluation of only one lung, some institutions routinely used median sternotomy even if there was no radiographic

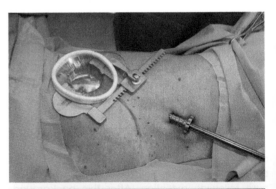

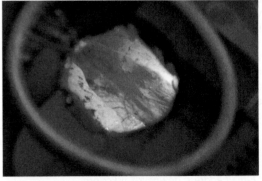

Fig. 2. Operative images of a left video-assisted muscle-sparing thoracotomy.

evidence for contralateral metastases. Retrospective series from such institutions suggested that occult disease would be found in the contralateral lung in approximately one-third of patients.[8] Concerns such as these raised two questions: whether the limited palpation of the lung available during minimally invasive techniques meant that gross disease would be unresected; and whether this would lead to a decrease in cure rates. The surgical field is clearly divided on whether palpation is necessary. In a survey of members of the European Society of Thoracic Surgeons, Internullo and coworkers[9] found that 65% consider bimanual palpation of the lung necessary, whereas 35% "consider it not always necessary" and 40% use VATS techniques with curative intent.

The question of completeness of resection was first addressed in a prospective single-arm published in 1996 in which patients first had VATS resection of all disease seen radiographically and palpitation, and then underwent thoracotomy with bimanual palpation of the lung.[10] Fifty-six percent of patients were found at thoracotomy to have sites of disease undetected at the time of VATS. Since then, questions have arisen about the applicability of these findings to a more modern practice because of improvements in minimally invasive surgery techniques and, more importantly, in computed tomography imaging. The results have proved durable. Multiple studies using modern technology have found similar results. For example, in 2011, Cerfolio and coauthors[11] published a prospective study of 152 patients undergoing thoracotomy and metastasectomy. Thirty patients had nodules palpated and resected that were not detected by computed tomography imaging. In a similar prospective study, Eckardt and Licht[12] found in 37 patients there were six metastases detected at thoracotomy after VATS resection of all radiographically evidence lesions. It is not clear from the manuscript how many of the 37 patients had additional lesions found, so the percentage of patients with additional metastases could range from 3% (one patient with 6 metastases out of 37) to 16% (six patients each with 1 additional metastasis out of 37).

The question that is more important is whether resection of the additional lesions found at thoracotomy translates into improved survival. This question has been recently addressed in a review article by Greenwood and West.[13] These authors found seven retrospective studies that compared long-term outcomes after VATS versus thoracotomy for metastasectomy. All seven studies found no significant difference in survival of patients undergoing either an open procedures or thoracoscopy.

Finally, research questions should be thoughtfully prioritized by importance given the time and expense involved in conducting prospective randomized trials. The question of how VATS techniques and open thoracotomy compare is interesting but less important than determining whether pulmonary metastasectomy by any technique improves survival over best medical therapies, and if so, determining the benefit according to histology of the primary disease and according to the tempo and burden of disease (ie, DFI and number of metastases).

POSTEROLATERAL THORACOTOMY

Posterolateral thoracotomy is probably the most commonly performed thoracotomy incision when wide exposure of a pleural space is needed. The first description is attributed by Curtis[14] to Nasiloff in 1888 in Russian, and the first English language description to Bryant in 1895. In turn, Curtis described a case report of a posterior thoracotomy performed in 1896 to retrieve an aspirated foreign body from the right lung, an effort involving two operations on consecutive days. In Europe, the incision is occasionally referred to as the "Craaford posterolateral thoracotomy" after the Swedish cardiothoracic surgeon[15]; the reason for this attribution is unclear.

In preparation for performing a posterolateral thoracotomy, the patient is positioned in the lateral decubitus position. A curvilinear incision is made from approximately two finger breadths lateral to the mid-spinal line, carried inferiorly and anteriorly to the tip of the scapula to the anterior axillary line. The latissimus muscle is most commonly completely divided, although descriptions of performing this incision by splitting the latissimus in the direction of its fibers have been published[15] (**Fig. 3**). The serratus anterior can

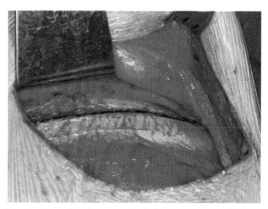

Fig. 3. Operative image of a right posterolateral thoracotomy showing division of latissimus muscle and elevation of scapula to allow exposure of the fifth interspace.

usually be mobilized and retracted anteriorly without division. The chest is most commonly entered through the fifth intercostal space and a rib spreader inserted. Posterior rib division or resection can facilitate exposure, but is often not necessary. This incision offers the greatest ease of performing thorough palpation of the ipsilateral lung, which is commonly helpful for locating very small metastases. If a rib is not divided, rib fracture is common. Closure of the incision is performed by placement of pericostal sutures, and reapproximation with a running suture of the latissimus dorsi muscle.

MUSCLE-SPARING INCISIONS

In our practice, the most commonly performed muscle-sparing thoracotomy is a vertical thoracotomy, with a 4- to 5-cm skin incision starting at the inferior aspect of the axilla and the anterior border of the latissimus dorsi muscle. The latissimus is mobilized until it can be retracted posteriorly, and the serratus anterior divided in the direction of its fibers, sparing branches of the thoracodorsal nerve if possible. The chest is most commonly entered over the sixth rib. A thoracoscopy retractor and a Wound-Guard are placed. Excellent exposure of the hilar structures is afforded, and complete palpation of the lung parenchyma should be possible. The ribs are closed with either one or no pericostal sutures, and the serratus reapproximated with an absorbable suture. No sutures need be placed in the latissimus dorsi.

The muscle-sparing thoracotomy seems to lead to considerably less pain and better preservation of shoulder girdle function than a posterolateral thoracotomy, and there is evidence that a muscle-sparing thoracotomy and VATS incisions are likely equivalent. Aswad and coauthors[16] performed a retrospective of 298 patients undergoing either VATS or muscle-sparing thoracotomy for the performance of a lung lobectomy, and found that the operative time with muscle-sparing thoracotomy was shorter and hospital stay was shorter with VATS, but otherwise the major parameters, such as postoperative complications, disease-free survival, and overall survival, were not different. Shortcomings of muscle-sparing thoracotomy include first the common finding that access to the posterior mediastinum (eg, level 7 lymph nodes) and to the superior mediastinum (eg, level 4 nodes) can be limited; and second, that extension of the incision either superiorly or toward the inframammary fold does not significantly increase exposure if needed (eg, to control bleeding).

MEDIAN STERNOTOMY

The first description of a median sternotomy was by Milton in 1897[17] and was performed to allow resection of anterior mediastinal masses. A median sternotomy offers excellent exposure to the anterior mediastinal structures, such as the heart and great vessels, and so is most commonly used for cardiac procedures. Sufficient exposure to the right and left pleural spaces is obtained to allow nonanatomic bilateral pulmonary procedures, such as wedge resection, although anatomic resections, such as a lobectomy, can be challenging. A median sternotomy probably produces less pain than a posterolateral thoracotomy. A disadvantage is the risk of infection, which is only rarely seen with a posterolateral thoracotomy and if it does occur, far more readily resolved.

In performing a sternotomy, the patient is positioned supine. Both arms are positioned at the patient's side. Having the arms extended when the sternum is opened with a retractor is thought to risk a traction injury of the brachial plexus over the first rib; the objective basis for this concern is not known to the authors. A midline incision is made from the sternal notch up to the xiphoid process. The pectoral fascia is divided, the periosteum of the sternum scored with cautery, and the sternum divided with a power saw. Closure is performed most commonly with simple or figure-of-eight, and number 6 wires are commonly used in adults. Robicsek and colleagues[18] have published a description of a lateral sternal wire weave that reinforces the sternum and costal margin for a more stable closure. Most often, two wires are placed in the manubrium and four in the body of the sternum. The pectoralis fascia is then approximated over the wires.

EXTENDED INCISIONS
Clamshell Thoracotomy

The vernacular term clamshell incision is technically described as a "transverse sternotomy with bilateral anterior thoracotomies."[19] Alternate names are a crossbow incision or transsternal bilateral thoracotomies. This approach was used frequently in the early years of cardiac surgery.[20–22] As median sternotomy became more popular for cardiac procedures, the use of the clamshell thoracotomy fell into disuse until the access afforded to the bilateral hila needed during bilateral lung transplants revived interest.[23]

The clamshell incision is performed with the patient supine, with the arms either flexed to 90° and secured to the ether screen, or extended laterally

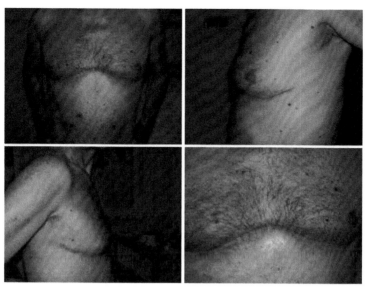

Fig. 4. Postoperative views after a clamshell thoracotomy.

on arm boards. The skin is incised along both infra-mammary creases. The pectoralis muscles are elevated bilaterally, with care being taken to leave a rim of muscle attached inferiorly on the chest wall to facilitate reattachment. Usually for resection of metastases, the chest is entered through the fourth interspace. The internal mammary vessels are ligated and divided bilaterally, and a transverse sternotomy performed. Retractors are placed. Access to the lung may be facilitated by single lung ventilation, and with division of the inferior pulmonary ligaments. The exposure is limited; it is most often of the left lower lobe of the lung. Obtaining wide exposure can also be problematic in women with large breasts because these need to be pushed cephalad from the level of the inframammary fold to the level of the fourth intercostal space. At the time of closure, bilateral chest tubes are placed and the sternum approximated with sternal wires, with the placement of a Steinmann pin bridging the upper

and lower aspects of the sternotomy to minimize the risk of overriding. The ribs are approximated using pericostal sutures, and the pectoralis muscle sewn to the chest wall. The procedure is well tolerated, although anecdotally patients note more often a sensation of chest stiffness or tightness with breathing than with a posterior lateral thoracotomy or a median sternotomy (**Fig. 4**).

Hemiclamshell Thoracotomy

A hemiclamshell incision combines a median sternotomy with a unilateral anterior thoracotomy and allows exposure of one lung and the structures of the mediastinum. It is most often performed for mediastinal tumors (eg, thymomas or germ cell tumors) extending into one pleural space, or for pulmonary malignancies invading the mediastinum; in our experience, it is rarely appropriate for resection of pulmonary metastases (**Table 1**).

Table 1
Summary of surgical approaches to resection of bilateral pulmonary metastases

Surgical Approach	Advantages	Disadvantages
Staged bilateral thoracotomies	Allows time for pathologic diagnosis; respiratory compromise limited to one lung	Two procedures and two hospitalizations
Simultaneous bilateral thoracotomies	One procedure and hospitalization	Most painful and most respiratory compromise
Median sternotomy	Bilateral exposure; less painful	Poor exposure to posterior lung fields
Clamshell thoracotomy	Excellent bilateral exposure	Sacrifice of both internal mammary arteries

REFERENCES

1. Edwards AT. Malignant disease of the lung. J Thorac Surg 1934;4:107–24.
2. Alexander J, Haight C. Pulmonary resection for solitary metastatic sarcoma and carcinomas. Surg Gynecol Obstet 1947;85:129–46.
3. Marcove RC, Mike V, Hajek JV, et al. Osteogenic sarcoma under the age of 21: a review of 145 operative cases. J Bone Joint Surg 1970;52A:411–21.
4. Martini N, Huvos AG, Mike V, et al. Multiple pulmonary resections in the treatment of osteogenic sarcoma. Ann Thorac Surg 1971;12:271–80.
5. Pastorino U, Buyse M, Friedel G, et al. Long-term results of lung metastasectomy: prognostic analyses based on 5206 cases. The International Registry of Lung Metastases. J Thorac Cardiovasc Surg 1997;113:37–49.
6. Migliore M, Milošević M, Lees B, et al. Finding the evidence for pulmonary metastasectomy in colorectal cancer: the PulMicc trial. Future Oncol 2015;11(2 Suppl):15–8.
7. Downey RJ, McCormack P, LoCicero J. 3rd Dissemination of malignant tumors after video-assisted thoracic surgery: a report of twenty-one cases. The Video-Assisted Thoracic Surgery Study Group. J Thorac Cardiovasc Surg 1996;111:954–60.
8. Roth JA, Pass HI, Wesley MN, et al. Comparison of median sternotomy and thoracotomy for resection of pulmonary metastases in patients with adult soft-tissue sarcomas. Ann Thorac Surg 1986;42:134–8.
9. Internullo E, Cassivi SD, Van Raemdonck D, et al. Treasure T on behalf of the ESTS Pulmonary Metastasectomy Working Group. Pulmonary metastasectomy: a survey of current practice amongst members of the European Society of Thoracic Surgeons. J Thorac Oncol 2008;3:1257–66.
10. McCormack PM, Bains MS, Begg CB, et al. Role of video-assisted thoracic surgery in the treatment of pulmonary metastases: results of a prospective trial. Ann Thorac Surg 1996;62(1):213–6.
11. Cerfolio RJ, McCarty T, Bryant AS. Non-imaged pulmonary nodules discovered during thoracotomy for metastasectomy by lung palpation. Eur J Cardiothorac Surg 2009;35:786–91.
12. Eckardt J, Licht PB. Thoracoscopic versus open pulmonary metastasectomy. A prospective, sequentially controlled study. Chest 2012;142(6):1598–602.
13. Greenwood A, West D. Is a thoracotomy rather than thoracoscopy resection associated with improved survival after pulmonary metastasectomy? Interact CardioVasc Thorac Surg 2013;17:720–4.
14. Curtis BF. Posterior thoracotomy for foreign body in the right bronchus. Ann Surg 1989;28(5):605.
15. Bellamy J, Santillan D. A new technique of posterolateral thoracotomy with preservation of the latissimus dorsi muscle. Ann Chir 1993;47(2):174–8.
16. Aswad BI, Jones RN, Kuritzky AM, et al. Lobectomy by video-assisted thoracic surgery vs muscle-sparing thoracotomy for stage I lung cancer: a critical evaluation of short- and long-term outcomes. J Am Coll Surg 2015;220:1044–53.
17. Milton H. Mediastinal surgery. Lancet 1897;1:872–5.
18. Robiscek F, Daugherty HK, Cook JW. The prevention and treatment of sternum separation following open-heart surgery. J Thorac Cardiovasc Surg 1977;73:267–8.
19. Bains MS, Ginsberg RG, Jones G II, et al. The clamshell incision: an improved approach to bilateral pulmonary and mediastinal tumors. Ann Thorac Surg 1994;58:30–3.
20. Johnson J, Kirby CK. Bilateral transpleural exposure of the heart. In: Johnson J, Kirby CK, editors. A handbook of operative surgery – surgery of the chest. Chicago: Year Book; 1958. p. 130–1.
21. Dobell ARC. Thoracic incisions. In: Sabiston DC, Spencer FC, editors. Gibbons surgery of the chest. 3rd edition. Philadelphia: WB Saunders; 1976. p. 146–59.
22. Bloomer WE. Thoracic incisions. In: Glenn WWL, editor. Thoracic and cardiovascular surgery. 4th edition. Norwalk (CT): Appleton-Century-Crofts; 1978. p. 103–4.
23. Egan TM, Detterbeck FC. Technique and results of double lung transplantation. Chest Surg Clin N Am 1993;3:89–111.

Ablative Approaches for Pulmonary Metastases

Matthew J. Boyer, MD, PhD[a], Umberto Ricardi, MD[b], David Ball, MB BS, MD, FRANZCR[c,d], Joseph K. Salama, MD[a,*]

KEYWORDS

- Pulmonary metastases • Ablative therapy • Radiotherapy • Oligometastases

KEY POINTS

- Directed treatment of pulmonary metastases was traditionally limited to surgical resection in appropriately selected patients.
- More recently, for patients who are not surgical candidates, non-invasive approaches such as radiotherapy or radiofrequency or microwave ablation have been developed.
- These techniques can provide local control and survival benefit similar to that seen with surgery in well selected patients, such as those with oligometastatic disease.
- Further studies are needed to define the role of ablative therapies compared to surgical management and the integration of these techniques with systemic treatments.

INTRODUCTION

Pulmonary metastases are a common event in patients with cancer. Approximately 50% of patients with malignancy-related deaths were found to have metastases in their lungs at autopsy.[1] This proclivity seems to involve tumor intrinsic factors including epidermal growth factor receptor (EGFR) signaling and matrix metalloproteinase expression, and unidentified factors present in the lung microenvironment.[2] Traditionally, systemic therapies including cytotoxic chemotherapy, hormonal therapies, immune-modulating therapy, monoclonal antibodies, and other "targeted" agents have been used to treat lung metastases. The role of ablative treatments directed at clinically evident metastases has been primarily limited to surgical resection in medically fit patients with long disease-free intervals and a minimal burden of systemic disease.[3] Based on the long history of surgical removal of pulmonary metastases,[4] and the combined diagnostic and therapeutic nature of the procedure, surgery is considered the standard approach for these patients. However, a significant number of patients are not candidates for metastasectomy, whether because of technically unresectable tumors, medical comorbidity rendering them unfit for surgery, a shorter disease-free interval, or extensive extrathoracic disease. For these patients, noninvasive or minimally invasive approaches to ablate pulmonary metastases are potential treatment strategies. This article discusses the data behind nonsurgical ablative approaches, namely ablative radiotherapy (stereotactic body radiation therapy [SBRT]) or thermal ablation via radiofrequency ablation (RFA) or microwave ablation (MWA), for pulmonary metastases.

[a] Department of Radiation Oncology, Duke University, Box 3085 DUMC, Durham, NC 27710, USA; [b] Department of Oncology, University of Turin, Regione Gonzole 10, 10043 Orbassano, Turin, Italy; [c] Department of Radiation Oncology, Peter MacCallum Cancer Centre, 2 St Andrews Pl, Melbourne, Victoria 3002, Australia; [d] The Sir Peter MacCallum Department of Oncology, The University of Melbourne, Parkville, Victoria 3010, Australia
* Corresponding author. Duke University Medical Center, Box 3085, Durham, NC 27710.
E-mail address: joseph.salama@duke.edu

Thorac Surg Clin 26 (2016) 19–34
http://dx.doi.org/10.1016/j.thorsurg.2015.09.004

BACKGROUND

Surgical resection of pulmonary metastases was described as early as the mid to late nineteenth century, likely because of advances in anesthesia and aseptic techniques.[4] The use of other metastasis-directed therapies, such as radiotherapy and invasive ablative techniques, has been developed more recently.[5] The use of metastasis-directed therapy techniques including surgery,[6] radiotherapy,[7] and invasive ablative strategies[8] has been increasing, likely mirroring the increasing use and availability of advanced imaging, such as high-resolution computed tomography (CT), MRI, and PET-CT to detect metastases when they are few in number and clinically asymptomatic. Furthermore, the increasing availability of advanced CT simulation techniques including multiplanar CT simulation, tumor-associated respiratory motion assessment, and respiratory motion management, and linear accelerators with associated image guidance, rapid dose delivery, and conformal therapy, make these techniques increasingly attractive tools for physicians and patients.

Additionally, a greater acceptance of the philosophic underpinnings of the use of metastasis-directed therapies is also contributing to their increasing use. The oligometastatic state was proposed by Hellman and Weichselbaum[9] as a distinct biologic state between locoregionally confined tumors and widespread metastatic disease. Based on the spectrum theory of cancer metastases,[10] oligometastases are metastases limited in number and destination organ, which in certain circumstances could represent disease unlikely to spread further. In this situation, metastasis-directed ablative therapies could improve the disease-free survival of patients by rendering them without evidence of cancer. Multiple studies consistently report about 25% long-term survival following metastasis-directed therapy to pulmonary (and other) metastases.[3,11,12]

Recent studies are beginning to describe the biology of the oligometastatic state. MicroRNA analyses of primary tumors and metastases undergoing ablative radiotherapy[13] and surgically resected pulmonary metastases[14] have demonstrated that specific microRNA expression patterns are associated with long-term disease control. Furthermore, when these microRNAs are overexpressed in murine models, a change in phenotype from oligometastasis to polymetastasis is observed. Regulation of oligometastases has been proposed to be controlled at some level by microRNA found on chromosome 14q32. These microRNAs suppressed cellular adhesion and invasion and inhibited metastasis development in an animal model of breast cancer lung colonization. Their target genes, including TGFBR2 and ROCK2, are thought to be key mediators of these effects.[15]

Greater biologic understanding of oligometastases raises some interesting questions regarding the use of ablative therapies. If biology truly governs the ability of these tumors to spread, then perhaps patients with oligometastases are destined to do well, and metastasis-directed ablative therapies might not be needed. Although analyses of patients with oligometastases who undergo ablative therapies for pulmonary metastases report better than expected outcomes, few reports have control groups of similar patients who have not received metastasis-directed therapy. Of the few that do, often no difference in overall survival is seen.[16] Ongoing randomized studies will help to determine if survival, or progression-free survival, is improved in patients receiving ablative therapies.

Role of Ablative Therapies

Although most attention has focused on the use of ablative techniques to improve survival in patients with pulmonary oligometastases, there are other clinical situations where these techniques are useful management strategies. In patients who are not candidates for or are unwilling to undergo systemic therapy, ablative therapies can be used as noninvasive or minimally invasive methods to halt the growth of metastases. This is also true for patients who have been on systemic therapy, but are not able to continue based on cumulative toxicity. Furthermore, in patients with polymetastases, a limited number of metastases may be growing while others lesions in the same patient may be stable on systemic therapy. This phenomenon, termed oligoprogression, has been described most clearly in patients with non–small cell lung cancer (NSCLC) with driver mutations treated with targeted therapies to EGFR mutations or ALK and ROS mutations. In oligoprogressive patients, the use of ablative techniques directed toward the few metastases, both intracranial and extracranial, that were progressing through targeted therapy prolonged the time that patients were able to stay on therapy and this directly improved survival because patients on targeted therapy longer than 2 years lived longer than those who were not.[17,18]

General Principles of Ablative Therapies

There are some common themes that permeate the literature regarding ablative therapies for pulmonary and extrapulmonary metastases. Perhaps most important is the emphasis placed on patient selection. Although approximately 25% of patients have long-term disease control following ablative therapies, 75% do not. The usual time to development of new metastases is only 6 months for patients undergoing ablative radiotherapy[19] and patients should be counseled regarding this. Patients with longer disease-free intervals from time of locoregional disease to development of metastases tend to have longer progression-free survival following ablative therapies.[3,11] Furthermore, patients with fewer metastases,[19] nonsynchronous presentation,[20] and those with metastases not progressing immediately before ablative therapies have improved outcomes.[21] For patients with breast cancer, those with estrogen receptor–positive tumors tend to do better than those with estrogen receptor–negative tumors.[21] Additionally, patients who are able to undergo a complete ablation/resection do better than those with incomplete resection.[3,21] All of these factors should be considered when recommending a patient for an ablative therapy for pulmonary metastases.

ABLATIVE RADIOTHERAPY FOR PULMONARY METASTASES
Background

Traditionally, radiation therapy for lung metastases has been limited to palliation of symptoms, such as cough, hemoptysis, dyspnea, or pain. Many radiation dose-fractionation schedules are currently used for palliation of thoracic symptoms, including 50 Gy in 25 fractions, 30 Gy in 10 fractions, 20 Gy in five fractions, and 17 Gy in two fractions, all of which have demonstrated approximately equal palliation and disease control compared with 10 Gy in a single fraction.[22] Although these regimens have demonstrated efficacy in short-term symptom management for patients with high burdens of disease and short life expectancy, they were never designed for long-term disease control, and durable treated tumor control is lacking.

The ability to deliver a larger biologically equivalent dose (BED) to ablate a targeted tumor over an equally short time period as palliative regimens, via larger daily doses, conformally "wrapped" around pulmonary metastases, has more recently become possible. This technique has been termed SBRT or stereotactic ablative radiotherapy, but it is best described as hypofractionated image-guided radiation therapy.[23] This treatment technique is a natural development following the success of intracranial radiosurgery

pioneered by Lars Leksell in the 1950s. Dr Leksell developed the technique of using a rigid frame affixed directly to the skull that could be used to create a coordinate system surrounding the head. This coordinate system could then be used to target lesions in the brain stereotactically to treat intracranial metastases with a single large dose that has been shown to achieve excellent control rates.[24] Low, acceptable rates of acute and late toxicity are seen with this technique because of sharp drop off of radiation dose between tumor targets and surrounding normal tissues. In essence, all of the tissue within the target receives a high dose of radiation and is ablated, whereas excluded surrounding normal tissue is spared.

Exporting this technique to extracranial targets presented significant challenges, only recently overcome, including accounting of respiratory-induced tumor motion, immobilization of the body that unlike the brain is not surrounded by a rigid skull, imaging techniques to precisely target tumors while patients are in the treatment position, radiotherapy planning algorithms to calculate dose extremely precisely, and linear accelerator treatment machines that have the mechanical capability to deliver these doses rapidly and precisely. Ablative radiotherapy treatments were preliminarily extended about a decade ago to primary early stage NSCLC not amenable to surgery with the well referenced Radiation Therapy Oncology Group (RTOG) 0236 trial by Timmerman and colleagues[25] demonstrating local control rates of greater than 90% (and comparable with surgery) serving as a standard for future studies.

It is hypothesized that this greater clinical control is caused by increased double-strand DNA breaks within the tumor cells themselves and disruption of the tumor microenvironment, notably the microvasculature, which is generally thought to be radioresistant at lower daily doses. There are data to suggest that endothelial cells undergo apoptosis after a threshold of 8 to 10 Gy with increasing cellular death up to 25 Gy[26] and that this may underlie the response to ablative radiotherapy.[27] A more recent study, however, showed that deletion of the proapoptotic gene *Bax* from endothelial cells did not alter the response of primary sarcomas to ablative doses of radiation.[28] Conversely, deletion of *Atm* from the sarcoma cells themselves did enhance tumor eradication.[28] Indeed the greater efficacy of ablative radiotherapy compared with conventionally fractionated treatment may merely be caused by the higher BED as predicted by the traditional linear-quadratic model of cellular death in response to radiation.[29]

Technical Aspects

Ablative radiotherapy is a technically precise treatment requiring the combination of many advances in radiation planning and delivery to achieve desired results[23] demonstrated for a patient with a pulmonary metastasis from head and neck cancer in **Fig. 1**. Early studies of SBRT used immobilization systems similar to intracranial stereotactic radiation.[5] However, similar to the advent of frameless intracranial radiosurgery, current courses of ablative radiotherapy are commonly planned and delivered with image guidance directly comparing cone beam, kilovoltage, or megavoltage CTs acquired on board the actual treatment delivery machine with the CT scans acquired at the time of simulation for treatment as shown in **Fig. 2**. Alternatively, implanted fiducial markers can be used for tumor targeting using orthogonal kilovoltage images. To achieve the needed set-up precision, patients are typically positioned supine with their arms above their head in a customized immobilization device created at the time of simulation. However, some systems do not require external patient immobilization and rely only on internal tumor tracking. Given the need for precise tumor targeting, knowledge of tumor motion is critical. A common way to determine this is via four-dimensional treatment planning CTs, which can depict the amount of tumor motion during the respiratory cycle. Based on the degree of motion observed, treatment is delivered either with free-breathing or with a respiratory motion management strategy. Typical respiratory motion management strategies include having the patient holding their breath during radiation treatment (typically in deep inspiration), active breathing control (where the patient's respiratory cycle is fixed via an external system), use of abdominal compression (minimizing diaphragm respiratory excursion), or with certain treatment machines delivery of radiation synchronized to specific phases of the respiratory cycle.[30]

Planning for ablative radiation involves contouring the targets on each slice of the axial CT images obtained at the time of simulation. The gross tumor volume consists of the known macroscopic disease, based on all available clinical, radiographic,

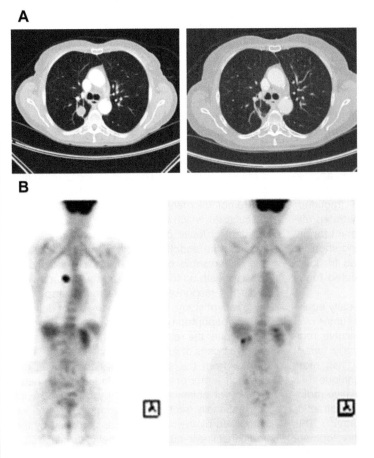

Fig. 1. Preablative and postablative radiotherapy CT (*A*) and PET (*B*) images showing a metastasis from head and neck squamous cell carcinoma completely resolving radiographically and metabolically.

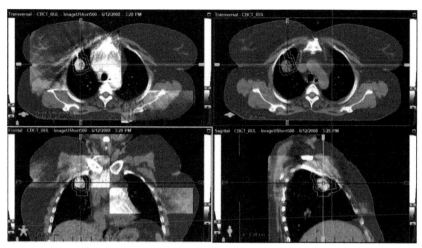

Fig. 2. Overlay of the planning CT and cone beam CT acquired at the time of each treatment. Note that the target volume in the axial, coronal, and sagittal planes contoured on the treatment planning CT fully encompasses the tumor visualized on the cone beam CT scan taken immediately before delivery of ablative radiotherapy while the patient is in the treatment position on the linear accelerator.

and metabolic information. The internal target volume is then created based on the amount of tumor movement visualized because of respiration. Finally, a 3- to 5-mm margin is placed on the internal target volume to create the planning target volume accounting for set-up uncertainty. Different from conventionally fractionated radiation therapy, no margin is added for microscopic tumor extension. Microscopic disease extension from the radiographically visible metastasis is encompassed in the radiation dose drop-off, which should control the lower density of tumor cells. Based on this volume and the dose to be delivered, and the nearby normal tissue and their respective dose constraints, a treatment plan is generated to produce a conformal dose distribution throughout the planning target volume while sparing surrounding healthy tissues. This can be achieved by several radiation delivery techniques including three-dimensional conformal therapy; intensity-modulated radiation therapy through a bouquet of multiple coplanar and noncoplanar fields; or volumetric-modulated arc therapy, which, when combined with image guidance before the delivery of each daily treatment, allow for precise and safe delivery of conformal, high dose per fraction treatment. In the case of three-dimensional conformal fixed-beam arrangements, it is preferable to use several beams (>8), some noncoplanar, which intersect only at the locus of the target, so that each beam contributes only a small dose to the surrounding normal tissues.

The optimal ablative radiation dose that maximizes tumor control while minimizing toxicity is unknown. Radiation doses used for pulmonary metastases are mostly the same as those used to treat early stage primary NSCLC, because both of these tumors were included in the early studies of pulmonary ablative radiotherapy. Practically, tumor size, location, and the patient's ability to tolerate treatment, and other logistic factors are considered when determining total dose and fractionation. Some studies have suggested that a BED higher than 100 Gy (ie, the dose at which tumor control is equal to 50 2-Gy fractions) is the minimum dose needed to control primary lung tumors and pulmonary metastases.[31,32] For three fraction regimens it seems that a dose of 54 Gy is necessary in pulmonary and hepatic tumors to achieve optimal control.[33] However, some regimens lower than the 100 Gy BED level have shown high rates of tumor control with limited toxicity and are frequently used in clinical practice.[34]

Pulmonary metastases often are located peripherally, spherical in shape, and contrast radiographically to surrounding lung tissue. Smaller metastases in the peripheral lung (ie, not within 2 cm of the bronchial tree) can generally be treated to higher doses with fewer fractions, including a single fraction. The phase II trial RTOG 0915 has completed accrual of patients with early stage medically inoperable NSCLC randomized to either 34 Gy in one fraction or 48 Gy total in four fractions. The 34-Gy single fraction arm had fewer adverse events and equivalent primary tumor control[35] and was planned to be compared with 54-Gy total in three fractions (based on RTOG 0236) but this comparison is not moving forward in the cooperative group setting. However, it is clear that single-fraction lung ablative radiosurgery to 26 to

30 Gy has been shown to be safe and effective in appropriately selected patients and tumor locations.[36] The ongoing SAFRON II trial (TROG 13.01 NCT01965223) is currently comparing single-dose 28 Gy to 48 Gy in four, 12-Gy fractions, specifically in the setting of pulmonary metastases. Because increased rates of grade 4 to 5 toxicity have been seen in patients treated with ablative radiotherapy to primary central tumors[37] (defined as within 2 cm of the bronchial tree or <1 cm away from major mediastinal blood vessels) alternative dosing strategies are needed for treatment to this region. RTOG 0813, a dose escalation study, is underway to determine the maximally tolerated dose for primary NSCLC tumors in this region. Alternatively, other risk-adapted radiation dosing strategies have been implemented incorporating a BED greater than 100 Gy in a slightly more fractionated schedule. One such strategy originating from Vrije Universiteit Amsterdam, delivering 60 Gy in eight 7.5-Gy fractions, has demonstrated treated tumor control rates (for centrally located, early stage NSCLC) equivalent to those achieved with three fraction regimens with acute and late toxicity profiles similar to those of peripheral lesions.[38]

Clinical Results

One of the first studies to investigate ablative radiotherapy for the treatment of pulmonary tumors included primary and metastatic tumors. A total of 22 out of 45 patients in this study had pulmonary metastases.[39] With a median follow-up of 11 months after treatment to 30 to 75 Gy in 5 to 10 fractions, overall treated tumor control was high at 97%. These and other promising early results[5] led to studies evaluating the use of ablative techniques specifically for pulmonary metastasis. A landmark multi-institutional dose-escalation study of 38 patients undergoing a three-fraction ablative regimen confirmed a 2-year treated metastasis control rate of 96%.[40] As summarized in **Table 1**, several other series have been reported (often combining primary and metastatic lung tumors) showing excellent tumor control with significant 1- and 2-year overall survival. Care must be taken in interpreting these data because of possible selection bias for those patients undergoing radiation therapy.

Ablative radiation has demonstrated efficacy for pulmonary metastases of many different histologies as shown in **Table 2**. These include sarcoma,[41] renal cell carcinoma,[42] melanoma, and colorectal[43] and gynecologic[19] malignancies. Although some of these histologies have historically been considered to be "radioresistant," no

tumors have been shown to be resistant to ablative radiotherapy. Although some series suggest that certain histologies are associated with worse treated tumor control and survival,[44] others series have not found histology to be an important determinant of tumor control.[33,45] Even for larger metastases, ablative radiation has demonstrated high rates of treated metastasis control with acceptable toxicity. Some analyses suggest that larger tumors are associated with worse treated metastasis control.[33] However in a cohort of patients treated with either 50 Gy in 10 fractions or with escalating doses of a three-fraction regimen, higher rates of treated tumor control were associated with treatment to at least 36 Gy in three fractions.[46] Overall, across many studies, 2-year treated metastasis control is of the order of 70% to 90%, which is comparable with pulmonary metastasectomy. Although these treatment modalities have not been prospectively compared directly, a retrospective comparison was published by Yu and colleagues[47] in 2014 that included 58 patients with metastatic osteosarcoma. Twenty-seven underwent SBRT to 70 Gy in seven fractions, whereas the remaining 31 underwent resection. Overall survival was approximately 40% in both groups. Similarly Widder and colleagues[48] showed a 3-year survival of 41% for metastasectomy and 49% for ablative radiotherapy in a retrospective review on 110 patients.

The treatment of multiple pulmonary metastases in the same treatment course is possible with ablative radiotherapy as shown in **Fig. 3**. In the previously mentioned landmark study by Rusthoven and colleagues,[40] the median number of treated metastases was two. Furthermore, studies evaluating the delivery of ablative radiotherapy to all known sites of metastases included patients with multiple pulmonary metastases, although the median number of metastases in these studies was also two.[19,49] However, despite this, treatment of more than two metastases in the same treatment course is technically challenging to ensure that radiation beams being used to target one metastasis do not overlap with those being used to treat another. If the beams being used to treat different metastases do overlap, they must be delivered on the same day to ensure that each metastasis receives the appropriate biologic dose. Furthermore, the dose from all treated pulmonary metastases must be summed to evaluate the cumulative dose to nearby organs at risk.

The primary pattern of progression following a course of ablative radiotherapy to pulmonary metastases is the appearance of other metastases, mainly in the lungs. In patients with

Table 1
Single institution series of ablative radiotherapy for primary pulmonary malignancies and pulmonary metastases

Author, Year	Country	Patients Met/Total	Median Follow-up (Months)	Total Dose (Gy)	Fractions	Treated Metastasis Control	Overall Survival
Blomgren et al,[5] 1995	Sweden	5/31	8.2	40 (mean)	1–3	92% crude	11 mo (mean)
Uematsu et al,[39] 1998	Japan	22/45	11	30–75	5–15	97% for both	—
Wulf et al,[45] 2005	Germany	45/81	14	30–37.5	3	72% at 1 y	85% at 1 y
Le et al,[82] 2006	United States	12/32	18	15–30	1	58% at 1 y	56% at 1 y
Yoon et al,[83] 2006	South Korea	53/91	14	30–48	3–4	80% at years	None surviving at 2 y
Hamamoto et al,[84] 2010	Japan	10/62	14	48	4	25% at 2 y	86% at 2 y
Takeda et al,[44] 2011	Japan	35/217	15–29	50	5	82% at 2 y	None surviving at 2 y
Yamamoto et al,[85] 2014	Japan	37/201	35	45–60	3–15	Approximately 65% at 2 y	Not reported
Davis et al,[86] 2015	United States and Germany	64/111	17	16–60	1–5	69.8% at 2 y	49.6% at 2 y

Data from Refs. 5,39,44,45,82–86

Table 2
Retrospective series of ablative radiotherapy for pulmonary metastases

Author, Year	Country	Patients	Median Follow-up (Months)	Total Dose (Gy)	Fractions	Treated Metastasis Control	Overall Survival
Okunieff et al,[34] 2006	United States	30	18.7	50–55	10	91% at 3 y	38% at 2 y
Norihisa et al,[32] 2008	Japan	34	27	48–60	4–5	90% at 2 y	84.3% at 2 y
Rusthoven et al,[40] 2009	United States	38	15.4	48–60	3	96% at 2 y	39% at 2 y
Zhang et al,[87] 2011	China	71	24.7	30–60	2–12	75.4% at 3 y	40.8% at 3 y
Ricardi et al,[88] 2012	Italy	61	20.4	26–45	1–4	89% at 2 y	66.5% at 2 y
Inoue et al,[89] 2013	Japan	87	15.4	48–60	4–10	80% at 3 y	32% at 3 y
Osti et al,[90] 2013	Italy	66	15	23–30	1	82.1% at 2 y	31.2% at 2 y
Filippi et al,[36] 2014	Italy	67	24	26	1	88.1% at 2 y	70.5% at 2 y
Singh et al,[91] 2014	United States	34	16.7	40–60	5	80% at 3 y	23% at 3 y
Garcia-Cabezas et al,[92] 2015	Spain	44	13.3	50–60	5–10	86.7% at 2 y	60.4% at 2 y
Navarria et al,[93] 2015	Italy	28	21	30–60	1–8	96% at 5 y	60.5% at 5 y
Nuyttens et al,[94] 2015	Netherlands	30	36	30–60	1–7	90% at 1 y	38% at 4 y
Siva et al,[95] 2015	Australia	65	25.2	18–26/48–50	1/4–5	93% at 2 y	71% at 2 y
Wang et al,[52] 2015	China	95	17	30–60	1–5	87% at 3 y	61.3% at 2 y

Data from Refs.[32,34,36,40,52,88–95]

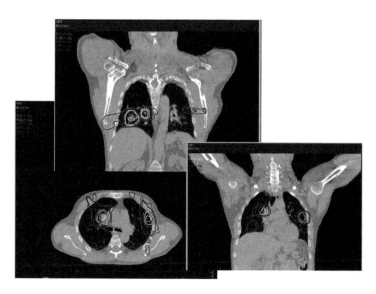

Fig. 3. Treatment planning CT of a patient with multiple synchronous lung metastases.

oligometastases treated with ablative radiotherapy to all known metastatic deposits, more than 50% of those whose disease progressed did so in a limited number of metastases.[30] Therefore, another course of metastasis-directed therapy might be appropriate. Multiple courses of ablative radiotherapy can be delivered for new metastases should it be clinically indicated,[50] similar to pulmonary metastasectomy.[3]

Toxicity

The organs at risk for pulmonary ablative radiotherapy include the lungs themselves, the chest wall and skin for peripherally located tumors, and the brachial plexus for apical lesions. The likelihood of toxicity seems to be correlated with the high-dose volume, tumor site (centrally vs peripherally located), and increasing size.[37] Fibrosis of the lung parenchyma is common after SBRT and manifests as an increased tissue density on CT in the area of the treated tumor, although it often does not give rise to clinically significant symptoms. Pulmonary function has been shown to be relatively preserved after ablative radiotherapy[51] but radiation pneumonitis and pneumonia have also been reported.[32,52] Increasing dose to normal lung seems to correlate with an increased incidence of pulmonary toxicity. The mean normalized total dose to the lung was shown to be 15 Gy in patients undergoing SBRT for multiple lung metastases with grade 2 or higher pulmonary toxicity compared with 8.5 Gy in those patients with no or grade 1 pulmonary toxicity.[53] This underscores the necessity to limit total lung dose, particularly in

the setting of treating multiple metastases, which inherently involves treating more normal lung tissue. When using intensity-modulated radiation therapy approaches where nontarget dose can be diffuse, it becomes important to limit the low-dose volumes using constraints, such as the volume of the contralateral lung receiving 5 Gy.

For peripherally located lung tumors the dose to the chest wall and skin must be considered. Rib fractures and chronic chest wall pain have also been observed after ablative radiotherapy.[36] Practically, grade 3 chest wall pain and rib fractures have been shown to occur when 30 mL or more of chest wall tissue within 3 cm of the lung/chest wall border received 30 Gy or higher in three to five fractions.[54] Alternatively 30 Gy to a volume of 70 mL of the chest wall defined as within 2 cm of the pleura was shown to be predictive of grade 2 or greater toxicity.[55] The risk of rib fracture is related to the total dose delivered to 2 mL of the rib.[56] Skin reactions are common with conventionally fractionated treatment and also need to be considered with SBRT. A report from MD Anderson showed a 10% risk for grade 2 or 3 dermatitis with 50 Gy total in four fractions to peripherally located tumors.[57] A single case of grade 4 necrosis has been reported.[58] Brachial plexopathy rises sharply after a maximum dose of 26 Gy in a single fraction indicating that this structure should be contoured and taken into account when treating apical metastases.[59] Despite this, high-grade toxicity is uncommon in series investigating ablative radiotherapy for pulmonary metastases, as noted in **Table 3**. Grade 3 or worse toxicity was seen in only a small percentage of patients.

Table 3
Toxicity in retrospective series presented in Table 2

Author, Year	Country	Patients	Grade 3 Toxicity or Greater	Comments
Okunieff et al,[34] 2006	United States	30	2%	1 patient with nonmalignant pleural effusion
Norihisa et al,[32] 2008	Japan	34	3%	1 patient required oxygen with pneumonia 18 months after treatment
Rusthoven et al,[40] 2009	United States	38	8%	3 patients, 1 pneumonitis, 1 rib fracture, 1 skin desquamation
Zhang et al,[87] 2011	China	71	0%	—
Ricardi et al,[88] 2012	Italy	61	1.6%	1 patient with pneumonitis
Inoue et al,[89] 2013	Japan	87	7%	1 patient with grade 4 pneumonitis
Osti et al,[90] 2013	Italy	66	3%	2 patients with pneumonitis
Filippi et al,[36] 2014	Italy	67	12% grade 2–3	2 rib fractures, 4 chronic chest wall pain
Singh et al,[91] 2014	United States	34	0%	—
Garcia-Cabezas et al,[92] 2015	Spain	44	0%	—
Navarria et al,[93] 2015	Italy	28	0%	—
Nuyttens et al,[94] 2015	Netherlands	30	10%	1 chronic pain, 1 fatigue, and 1 pneumonitis
Siva et al,[95] 2015	Australia	65	0%	—
Wang et al,[52] 2015	China	95	3.2%	3 patients with pneumonitis

Data from Refs.[32,34,36,40,52,87–95]

Combining Ablative Radiotherapy and Systemic Therapy

After SBRT for pulmonary metastases 46% to 77% of patients develop new sites of metastatic disease. This highlights the need for systemic therapy in addition to metastasis-directed ablative therapies for most patients. There are few data regarding the use or timing of cytotoxic chemotherapy with SBRT. Although it is commonly used concurrently or sequentially with conventionally fractionated radiotherapy, there is hesitation to prescribe systemic therapy together or immediately after ablative radiotherapy. In one study of patients with oligometastases, including but not limited to pulmonary malignancies, the maximum tolerated dose of sunitinib, a receptor tyrosine kinase inhibitor, was shown to be 37.5 mg daily when given concurrently with 50 Gy divided into 10 daily fractions with 4-year overall survival of 29%.[60] A small phase II study in 2014 demonstrated that erlotinib, an EGFR inhibitor, was well tolerated when combined with SBRT to multiple progressing sites of metastatic NSCLC, including the lung, with only two grade 3 toxicities reported. Progression-free survival was 14.6 months and overall survival was 20.4 months.[61] Interestingly, none of the 13 patients whose tumors underwent mutational analysis, out of a total of 24 in the study, harbored a known EGFR mutation.[61] This suggests there may be a synergistic effect of inhibition of signaling through the EGFR pathway when combined with ablative radiotherapy.

Ongoing Studies

Although the body of evidence describing the outcomes of patients treated with ablative radiotherapy for pulmonary metastases continues to grow, most studies are retrospective series from single institutions. Many prospective studies are ongoing to answer important questions regarding the use of these treatments for patients with pulmonary metastases. One such important question is a comparison of the effectiveness of ablative radiotherapy with conventionally fractionated radiation. The SPACE study (NCT Identifier: NCT01920789) investigated 70 Gy in 35 fractions versus 45 Gy in three fractions for early stage NSCLC and showed no difference in local control or survival between the arms at 3 years.[62] The CHISEL study (TROG 09.02, NCT Identifier: NCT01014130) comparing 60 Gy in 30 fractions or 66 Gy in 33 fractions or 66 Gy in 33 fractions versus 54 Gy in three fractions has completed accrual in patients with stage I NSCLC. Although the results of ablative doses of radiation are better than expected, these studies will help determine the magnitude of benefit, if any, over conventional radiation. It is possible that the better than historical outcomes seen with ablative techniques are because of other coincidently developed technologies, such as PET staging, better patient immobilization, four-dimensional planning, tumor tracking, and better radiation-planning algorithms, rather than the ablative doses themselves. Although ablative techniques have an inherent utility for some patients with metastases because of their short duration, this benefit of this logistical convenience should be validated for true benefit over conventionally fractionated radiotherapy.

Furthermore, for patients with oligometastases, the Stereotactic Ablative Radiotherapy for Comprehensive Treatment of Oligometastatic Tumors (SABR-COMET) study is randomizing patients with five or fewer metastatic lesions, including pulmonary metastases, to either standard of care systemic therapy and palliative radiation or ablative radiotherapy to identify a survival improvement. Pulmonary metastases in this study are treated to between 54 and 60 Gy in three to eight fractions based on location and potential for normal tissue toxicity. Additionally, NRG BR001 is a phase I dose de-escalation study attempting to identify the optimal ablative radiotherapy doses for patients with two anatomically close, or three or four extracranial metastases. In this study, pulmonary metastases are initially treated to 45 to 50 Gy in three to five fractions based on location with one step dose de-escalation should normal tissue toxicity develop. A second randomized phase II/III study, NRG BR002, which is limited to patients with breast cancer, is comparing systemic therapy with or without SBRT or surgical resection of all visualized extracranial metastases. The Conventional care Or Radioablation (SBRT) for Extracranial oligometastatic disease in lung, breast and prostate cancer (CORE) study, funded by Cancer Research UK is testing the feasibility of randomizing patients to standard care or standard care plus SBRT for up to three metastases.

RADIOFREQUENCY ABLATION
Technique

RFA uses an alternating electrical current of 400 to 500 kHz delivered to the target tissue via an interstitial probe. This current creates heat via oscillating ions, and when taken to temperatures greater than 60°C, coagulative necrosis results. Typical treatment duration is 12 to 15 minutes. Although more often used for ablation of hepatic tumors,[63] ablation of pulmonary tumors including metastases is increasingly performed. Regardless, the Food and Drug Administration recently issued a public health notification explicitly forbidding the marketing of RFA systems for the specific treatment of lung tumors.[64]

Similar to ablative radiation, tumor location in the lung must be accounted for in the planning of RFA because adjacent blood vessels can serve as a heat sink and tumors surrounded, and insulated, by air-filled lung parenchyma require less energy compared with lesions situated along the pleura.[61] Most commonly multiple electrodes are inserted into the treated tumor simultaneously through a single, expandable needle. Electrodes can be placed with conscious sedation under CT guidance. For more central lesions, open procedures under general anesthesia are required. It has been shown that CT-guided biopsy and ablation can be performed at the same time, thereby minimizing the number of invasive procedures and their associated risks.[65] However, biopsy-related bleeding sometimes makes it difficult to localize targets for placement of RFA electrodes.[66]

Outcomes

Treated tumor control after RFA is difficult to assess given the opacified appearance of treated lung tissue on chest imaging. Follow-up CT and selective PET imaging of primary lung tumors treated with RFA have revealed an incomplete ablation rate approaching 40%.[67,68] In a study of 20 patients in which 24 lesions were treated, hypermetabolic activity on PET 3 to 6 months after ablation, but not 1 to 2 weeks after ablation, was predictive of response.[69] Of the four sites with recurrence, the mean maximum standardized uptake value 3 to 6 months after treatment was significantly higher at 4.8 compared with 1.8 at those sites without recurrence. Factors that have been shown to correlate with inferior control following RFA include lesions greater than 2 to 3 cm[8,70,71] and location near a large blood vessel, which may act as a heat sink.[71] In a study of 32 tumors resected after RFA, only 37.5% demonstrated complete tumor cell necrosis.[72]

Overall survival and toxicity from several large series are summarized in **Table 4**. The largest study, by de Baere and colleagues,[8] reported a 5-year overall survival greater than 50%. However, the rate of pneumothoraces in these studies was high at approximately 30% with a significant percentage requiring intervention. Two single-arm prospective

Table 4
Outcomes of radiofrequency ablation for pulmonary metastases

Author, Year	Patients	Median Follow-up (Months)	Overall Survival	Toxicity
Yan et al,[96] 2006	55	24	64% at 2 y	Pneumothorax rate, 29.1%
Simon et al,[97] 2007	57	27.5	44% at 2 y	Pneumothorax rate, 28.4% Procedure-specific mortality, 2.6%
Lencioni et al,[74] 2008	73	Not reported	64% at 2 y	Pneumothorax rate, 25.5%
von Meyenfeldt et al,[77] 2011	90	22	69% at 3 y	Pneumothorax rate, 34%
Palussiere et al,[78] 2012	67	21.3	Median survival 26 mo	Pneumothorax rate, 36%
Petre et al,[98] 2013	45	18	50% at 3 y	Pneumothorax rate, 33%
Koelblinger et al,[99] 2014	22	20	51% at 3 y	Grade 3 toxicity in 6.6%
de Baere et al,[8] 2015	566	35.5	51.5% at 5 y	Pneumothorax requiring treatment in 39%

Data from Refs.[8,74,77,78,96–99]

trials have reported similar early results.[73,74] A total of 100 peripheral lung tumors in 60 patients with a mean size of 17 mm and standard deviation of 9 mm were treated with RFA at the Institut Gustave Roussy.[73] Fifty-one percent of patients had multiple synchronous tumors. The 18-month treated metastasis control, disease-free survival, and overall survival were 88%, 34%, and 71%, respectively. A pneumothorax was documented after 54% of the RFA procedures; 23% required aspiration and 9% required chest tube placement. No patients died from treatment-related toxicity. A similar multi-institutional study enrolled 105 patients with one to three primary or metastatic lung tumors for RFA; maximum allowed tumor diameter was 3.5 cm.[74] One hundred eighty-three tumors were treated and the mean number of tumors per patient was 1.7 (standard deviation, 1.3). At 1 year, the rate of treated metastasis control and overall survival were 88% and 70%, respectively. Pneumothorax requiring intervention occurred in 20% of the procedures; there were no treatment-related deaths.

No randomized studies comparing RFA, surgical resection, and/or ablative radiotherapy exist, nor are they likely to be undertaken. A retrospective study from Japan published this year compared patients with primary NSCLC less than 5 cm in diameter undergoing RFA at one institution with SBRT at a different institution.[75] With just under 50 patients per group, there was no difference in 3-year overall survival (86.4% vs 79.6%)

or treated metastasis progression (9.6% vs 7.0%) between RFA and SBRT, respectively, although the distant recurrence rate was significantly higher with RFA.[75] In a study of 116 patients undergoing sublobar resection, SBRT, or RFA for stage I NSCLC, overall survival was not significantly different among the groups.[76] However, compared with resection and when controlled for tumor size and patient age, RFA patients had a hazard ratio for primary tumor recurrence of 7.57, whereas that for SBRT was 2.73.[76]

A report of oligometastatic lung tumors treated with RFA was recently published. Forty-six patients with 90 metastases ablated by RFA were included with a median follow-up of 22 months.[77] Pneumothorax occurred in 34% of the procedures with 25% requiring chest tube placement. Actuarial ablated tumor control at 1 and 2 years was 78% and 65%, respectively, with two-thirds of recurrences happening within 12 months. Overall survival at 3 years was significantly worse for patients with incomplete tumor ablation (49% vs 79%).

Studies have also reported the ability to treat bilateral pulmonary oligometastases in a single session.[78] However, of the 67 patients with one to five accessible tumors less than 4 cm, only 27 of 67 patients successfully completed bilateral RFA. Of the 40 that did not, 24 developed pneumothoraces that precluded treatment of the contralateral lung. In the patients that were able to undergo bilateral RFA, there was a high rate of pneumothorax

(67%) with 12 patients (44%) requiring chest tube placement. Four patients developed bilateral pneumothoraces and four patients (15%) experienced recurrence at a median of 9.5 months after RFA.

MICROWAVE ABLATION

Similar to RFA, MWA causes tumor destruction via hyperthermia. However, different from RFA, MWA uses higher frequencies of 915 MHz to 2.45 GHz. This induces rapid heating caused by forced rotation of polar molecules, mostly water, leading to higher temperatures compared with RFA. MWA can heat treated tumors in about 2 to 5 minutes, which is faster than the 12 to 15 minutes typical of RFA.[79] As a newer modality, the data reporting the outcomes of patients with MWA are less robust than that for RFA, although given the comparable procedures and mechanism of action, they seem to be similar.[80,81] Both RFA and MWA may have a role in patients previously irradiated for whom further radiotherapy is relatively contraindicated.

SUMMARY

Pulmonary metastases are common in patients with metastatic cancer. Ablative therapy, via radiotherapy, RFA, or MWA, has the theoretic advantage over metastasectomy to be less invasive and more effective, because of lower morbidity rates, lower costs, and the potential for delivering ablative treatments on an outpatient basis. However, when treating patients with metastases, even if oligometastatic, selection criteria are a pivotal issue. In general, clinical indications are the same as those for metastasectomy, but without the limits regarding patients unfit for surgery. The introduction of the concept of oligometastases and the implementation of a powerful tool to ablate tumors in alternative or in combination with surgery might be the basis for a paradigm shift in patients with oligometastases, moving from a purely palliative scenario toward a more curative approach. More prospective controlled studies are needed in the next years to understand the real impact of this strategy on clinical outcomes, not only in terms of tumor control and clinical safety, but also real survival benefit. In addition, for patients with cancer that progresses, future studies should focus on comparison of these techniques or how they can integrate into systemic treatment of patients with metastatic cancer to the lungs.

REFERENCES

1. Abrams HL, Spiro R, Goldstein N. Metastases in carcinoma; analysis of 1000 autopsied cases. Cancer 1950;3(1):74–85.
2. Chiang AC, Massague J. Molecular basis of metastasis. N Engl J Med 2008;359(26):2814–23.
3. Pastorino U, Buyse M, Friedel G, et al, The International Registry of Lung Metastases. Long-term results of lung metastasectomy: prognostic analyses based on 5206 cases. J Thorac Cardiovasc Surg 1997;113(1):37–49.
4. Alexander J, Haight C. Pulmonary resection for solitary metastatic sarcomas and carcinomas. Surg Gynecol Obstet 1947;85:129–46.
5. Blomgren H, Lax I, Näslund I, et al. Stereotactic high dose fraction radiation therapy of extracranial tumors using an accelerator. Clinical experience of the first thirty-one patients. Acta Oncol 1995;34(6):861–70.
6. Bartlett EK, Simmons KD, Wachtel H, et al. The rise in metastasectomy across cancer types over the past decade. Cancer 2015;121(5):747–57.
7. Lewis SL, Porceddu S, Nakamura N, et al. Definitive stereotactic body radiotherapy (SBRT) for extracranial oligometastases: an international survey of >1000 radiation oncologists. Am J Clin Oncol 2015. [Epub ahead of print].
8. de Baere T, Aupérin A, Deschamps F, et al. Radiofrequency ablation is a valid treatment option for lung metastases: experience in 566 patients with 1037 metastases. Ann Oncol 2015;26(5):987–91.
9. Hellman S, Weichselbaum RR. Oligometastases. J Clin Oncol 1995;13(1):8–10.
10. Hellman S. Karnofsky Memorial Lecture. Natural history of small breast cancers. J Clin Oncol 1994;12(10):2229–34.
11. Fong Y, Cohen AM, Fortner JG, et al. Liver resection for colorectal metastases. J Clin Oncol 1997;15(3):938–46.
12. Tanvetyanon T, Robinson LA, Schell MJ, et al. Outcomes of adrenalectomy for isolated synchronous versus metachronous adrenal metastases in non-small-cell lung cancer: a systematic review and pooled analysis. J Clin Oncol 2008;26(7):1142–7.
13. Lussier YA, Xing HR, Salama JK, et al. MicroRNA expression characterizes oligometastasis(es). PLoS One 2011;6(12):e28650.
14. Lussier YA, Khodarev NN, Regan K, et al. Oligo- and polymetastatic progression in lung metastasis(es) patients is associated with specific microRNAs. PLoS One 2012;7(12):e50141.
15. Uppal A, Wightman SC, Mallon S, et al. 14q32-encoded microRNAs mediate an oligometastatic phenotype. Oncotarget 2015;6(6):3540–52.
16. Aberg T, Malmberg KA, Nilsson B, et al. The effect of metastasectomy: fact or fiction? Ann Thorac Surg 1980;30(4):378–84.
17. Gan GN, Weickhardt AJ, Scheier B, et al. Stereotactic radiation therapy can safely and durably control sites of extra-central nervous system oligoprogressive disease in anaplastic lymphoma kinase-

positive lung cancer patients receiving crizotinib. Int J Radiat Oncol Biol Phys 2014;88(4):892–8.

18. Weickhardt AJ, Scheier B, Burke JM, et al. Local ablative therapy of oligoprogressive disease prolongs disease control by tyrosine kinase inhibitors in oncogene-addicted non-small-cell lung cancer. J Thorac Oncol 2012;7(12):1807–14.

19. Salama JK, Hasselle MD, Chmura SJ, et al. Stereotactic body radiotherapy for multisite extracranial oligometastases: final report of a dose escalation trial in patients with 1 to 5 sites of metastatic disease. Cancer 2012;118(11):2962–70.

20. de Vin T, Engels B, Gevaert T, et al. Stereotactic radiotherapy for oligometastatic cancer: a prognostic model for survival. Ann Oncol 2014;25(2):467–71.

21. Abbott DE, Brouquet A, Mittendorf EA, et al. Resection of liver metastases from breast cancer: estrogen receptor status and response to chemotherapy before metastasectomy define outcome. Surgery 2012;151(5):710–6.

22. Bezjak A. Palliative therapy for lung cancer. Semin Surg Oncol 2003;21(2):138–47.

23. Kirkpatrick JP, Kelsey CR, Palta M, et al. Stereotactic body radiotherapy: a critical review for non-radiation oncologists. Cancer 2013;120(7):942–54.

24. Kocher M, Soffietti R, Abacioglu U, et al. Adjuvant whole-brain radiotherapy versus observation after radiosurgery or surgical resection of one to three cerebral metastases: results of the EORTC 22952-26001 study. J Clin Oncol 2011;29(2):134–41.

25. Timmerman R, Paulus R, Galvin J, et al. Stereotactic body radiation therapy for inoperable early stage lung cancer. JAMA 2010;303(11):1070–6.

26. Fuks Z, Kolesnick R. Engaging the vascular component of the tumor response. Cancer Cell 2005;8(2):89–91.

27. Truman JP, García-Barros M, Kaag M, et al. Endothelial membrane remodeling is obligate for anti-angiogenic radiosensitization during tumor radiosurgery. PLoS One 2010;5(8):e12310.

28. Moding EJ, Castle KD, Perez BA, et al. Tumor cells, but not endothelial cells, mediate eradication of primary sarcomas by stereotactic body radiation therapy. Sci Transl Med 2015;7(278):278ra34.

29. Brown JM, Carlson DJ, Brenner DJ. The tumor radiobiology of SRS and SBRT: are more than the 5 Rs involved? Int J Radiat Oncol Biol Phys 2014;88(2):254–62.

30. Salama JK, Kirkpatrick JP, Yin FF. Stereotactic body radiotherapy treatment of extracranial metastases. Nat Rev Clin Oncol 2012;9(11):654–65.

31. Guckenberger M, Wulf J, Mueller G, et al. Dose-response relationship for image-guided stereotactic body radiotherapy of pulmonary tumors: relevance of 4D dose calculation. Int J Radiat Oncol Biol Phys 2009;74(1):47–54.

32. Norihisa Y, Nagata Y, Takayama K, et al. Stereotactic body radiotherapy for oligometastatic lung tumors. Int J Radiat Oncol Biol Phys 2008;72(2):398–403.

33. McCammon R, Schefter TE, Gaspar LE, et al. Observation of a dose-control relationship for lung and liver tumors after stereotactic body radiation therapy. Int J Radiat Oncol Biol Phys 2009;73(1):112–8.

34. Okunieff P, Petersen AL, Philip A, et al. Stereotactic body radiation therapy (SBRT) for lung metastases. Acta Oncol 2006;45(7):808–17.

35. Videtic GM, Hu C, Singh A, et al. Radiation Therapy Oncology Group (RTOG) Protocol 0915: a randomized phase 2 study comparing 2 stereotactic body radiation therapy (SBRT) schedules for medically inoperable patients with stage I peripheral non-small cell lung cancer. Int J Radiat Oncol Biol Phys 2013;87(2):S3.

36. Filippi AR, Badellino S, Guarneri A, et al. Outcomes of single fraction stereotactic ablative radiotherapy for lung metastases. Technol Cancer Res Treat 2014;13(1):37–45.

37. Timmerman R, McGarry R, Yiannoutsos C, et al. Excessive toxicity when treating central tumors in a phase II study of stereotactic body radiation therapy for medically inoperable early-stage lung cancer. J Clin Oncol 2006;24(30):4833–9.

38. Haasbeek CJ, Lagerwaard FJ, Slotman BJ, et al. Outcomes of stereotactic ablative radiotherapy for centrally located early-stage lung cancer. J Thorac Oncol 2011;6(12):2036–43.

39. Uematsu M, Shioda A, Tahara K, et al. Focal, high dose, and fractionated modified stereotactic radiation therapy for lung carcinoma patients: a preliminary experience. Cancer 1998;82(6):1062–70.

40. Rusthoven KE, Kavanagh BD, Burri SH, et al. Multi-institutional phase I/II trial of stereotactic body radiation therapy for lung metastases. J Clin Oncol 2009;27(10):1579–84.

41. Dhakal S, Corbin KS, Milano MT, et al. Stereotactic body radiotherapy for pulmonary metastases from soft-tissue sarcomas: excellent local lesion control and improved patient survival. Int J Radiat Oncol Biol Phys 2012;82(2):940–5.

42. Ranck MC, Golden DW, Corbin KS, et al. Stereotactic body radiotherapy for the treatment of oligometastatic renal cell carcinoma. Am J Clin Oncol 2013;36(6):589–95.

43. Hoyer M, Roed H, Hansen AT, et al. Prospective study on stereotactic radiotherapy of limited-stage non-small-cell lung cancer. Int J Radiat Oncol Biols Phys 2006;66(4 Suppl):S128–35.

44. Takeda A, Kunieda E, Ohashi T, et al. Stereotactic body radiotherapy (SBRT) for oligometastatic lung tumors from colorectal cancer and other primary cancers in comparison with primary lung cancer. Radiother Oncol 2011;101(2):255–9.

45. Wulf J, Baier K, Mueller G, et al. Dose-response in stereotactic irradiation of lung tumors. Radiother Oncol 2005;77(1):83–7.

46. Corbin K, Ranck MC, Hasselle MD, et al. Feasibility and toxicity of hypofractionated image-guided radiotherapy for large volume limited metastatic disease. Pract Radiat Oncol 2013;3(4):316–22.

47. Yu W, Tang L, Lin F, et al. Stereotactic radiosurgery, a potential alternative treatment for pulmonary metastases from osteosarcoma. Int J Oncol 2014; 44(4):1091–8.

48. Widder J, Klinkenberg TJ, Ubbels JF, et al. Pulmonary oligometastases: metastasectomy or stereotactic ablative radiotherapy? Radiother Oncol 2013; 107(3):409–13.

49. Milano MT, Katz AW, Zhang H, et al. Oligometastases treated with stereotactic body radiotherapy: long-term follow-up of prospective study. Int J Radiat Oncol Biol Phys 2012;83(3):878–86.

50. Milano MT, Philip A, Okunieff P. Analysis of patients with oligometastases undergoing two or more curative-intent stereotactic radiotherapy courses. Int J Radiat Oncol Biol Phys 2009;73(3):832–7.

51. Stephans KL, Djemil T, Reddy CA, et al. Comprehensive analysis of pulmonary function Test (PFT) changes after stereotactic body radiotherapy (SBRT) for stage I lung cancer in medically inoperable patients. J Thorac Oncol 2009;4(7):838–44.

52. Wang Z, Kong QT, Li J, et al. Clinical outcomes of cyberknife stereotactic radiosurgery for lung metastases. J Thorac Dis 2015;7(3):407–12.

53. Yenice KM, Partouche J, Cunliffe A, et al. Analysis of radiation pneumonitis (RP) incidence in a phase I stereotactic body radiotherapy (SBRT) dose escalation study for multiple metastases. Int J Radiat Oncol Biol Phys 2010;78(3, Suppl):S25 [Abstract: 53].

54. Dunlap NE, Cai J, Biedermann GB, et al. Chest wall volume receiving >30 Gy predicts risk of severe pain and/or rib fracture after lung stereotactic body radiotherapy. Int J Radiat Oncol Biol Phys 2010;76(3): 796–801.

55. Mutter RW, Liu F, Abreu A, et al. Dose-volume parameters predict for the development of chest wall pain after stereotactic body radiation for lung cancer. Int J Radiat Oncol Biol Phys 2012;82(5): 1783–90.

56. Pettersson N, Nyman J, Johansson KA. Radiation-induced rib fractures after hypofractionated stereotactic body radiation therapy of non-small cell lung cancer: a dose- and volume-response analysis. Radiother Oncol 2009;91(3):360–8.

57. Welsh J, Thomas J, Shah D, et al. Obesity increases the risk of chest wall pain from thoracic stereotactic body radiation therapy. Int J Radiat Oncol Biol Phys 2011;81(1):91–6.

58. Hoppe BS, Laser B, Kowalski AV, et al. Acute skin toxicity following stereotactic body radiation therapy for stage I non-small-cell lung cancer: who's at risk? Int J Radiat Oncol Biol Phys 2008;72(5):1283–6.

59. Forquer JA, Fakiris AJ, Timmerman RD, et al. Brachial plexopathy from stereotactic body radiotherapy in early-stage NSCLC: dose-limiting toxicity in apical tumor sites. Radiother Oncol 2009;93(3): 408–13.

60. Kao J, Chen CT, Tong CC, et al. Concurrent sunitinib and stereotactic body radiotherapy for patients with oligometastases: final report of a prospective clinical trial. Target Oncol 2014;9(2):145–53.

61. Iyengar P, Kavanagh BD, Wardak Z, et al. Phase II trial of stereotactic body radiation therapy combined with erlotinib for patients with limited but progressive metastatic non-small-cell lung cancer. J Clin Oncol 2014;32(34):3824–30.

62. Nyman J, AH, Lund JA, et al. SPACE: a randomized study of SBRT vs conventional fractionated radiotherapy in medically inoperable stage I NSCLC. Proceeding of ESTRO 33. Vienna, Austria, April 4-8, 2014.

63. Curley SA, Izzo F, Delrio P, et al. Radiofrequency ablation of unresectable primary and metastatic hepatic malignancies: results in 123 patients. Ann Surg 1999;230(1):1–8.

64. US Food and Drug Administration. FDA public health notification: radiofrequency ablation of lung tumors: clarification of regulatory status. 2008. Available at: http://www.fda.gov/MedicalDevices/Safety/Alertsand Notices/PublicHealthNotifications/ucm061985.htm. Accessed October 6, 2015.

65. Schneider T, Puderbach M, Kunz J, et al. Simultaneous computed tomography-guided biopsy and radiofrequency ablation of solitary pulmonary malignancy in high-risk patients. Respiration 2012;84(6): 501–8.

66. Fernando HC. Radiofrequency ablation to treat non-small cell lung cancer and pulmonary metastases. Ann Thorac Surg 2008;85(2):S780–4.

67. Ambrogi MC, Fanucchi O, Cioni R, et al. Long-term results of radiofrequency ablation treatment of stage I non-small cell lung cancer: a prospective intention-to-treat study. J Thorac Oncol 2011;6(12):2044–51.

68. Fernando HC, De Hoyos A, Landreneau RJ, et al. Radiofrequency ablation for the treatment of non-small cell lung cancer in marginal surgical candidates. J Thorac Cardiovasc Surg 2005; 129(3):639–44.

69. Higuchi M, Honjo H, Shigihara T, et al. A phase II study of radiofrequency ablation therapy for thoracic malignancies with evaluation by FDG-PET. J Cancer Res Clin Oncol 2014;140(11):1957–63.

70. Lee JM, Jin GY, Goldberg SN, et al. Percutaneous radiofrequency ablation for inoperable non-small cell lung cancer and metastases: preliminary report. Radiology 2004;230(1):125–34.

71. Gillams AR, Lees WR. Radiofrequency ablation of lung metastases: factors influencing success. Eur Radiol 2008;18(4):672–7.

72. Schneider T, Reuss D, Warth A, et al. The efficacy of bipolar and multipolar radiofrequency ablation of lung neoplasms: results of an ablate and resect study. Eur J Cardiothorac Surg 2011;39(6):968–73.

73. de Baere T, Palussière J, Aupérin A, et al. Midterm local efficacy and survival after radiofrequency ablation of lung tumors with minimum follow-up of 1 year: prospective evaluation. Radiology 2006;240(2):587–96.

74. Lencioni R, Crocetti L, Cioni R, et al. Response to radiofrequency ablation of pulmonary tumours: a prospective, intention-to-treat, multicentre clinical trial (the RAPTURE study). Lancet Oncol 2008;9(7): 621–8.

75. Ochiai S, Yamakado K, Kodama H, et al. Comparison of therapeutic results from radiofrequency ablation and stereotactic body radiotherapy in solitary lung tumors measuring 5 cm or smaller. Int J Clin Oncol 2015;20(3):499–507.

76. Safi S, Rauch G, op den Winkel J, et al. Sublobar resection, radiofrequency ablation or radiotherapy in stage I non-small cell lung cancer. Respiration 2015;89(6):550–7.

77. von Meyenfeldt EM, Prevoo W, Peyrot D, et al. Local progression after radiofrequency ablation for pulmonary metastases. Cancer 2011;117(16):3781–7.

78. Palussiere J, Gómez F, Cannella M, et al. Single-session radiofrequency ablation of bilateral lung metastases. Cardiovasc Intervent Radiol 2012;35(4):852–9.

79. Smith SL, Jennings PE. Lung radiofrequency and microwave ablation: a review of indications, techniques and post-procedural imaging appearances. Br J Radiol 2015;88(1046):20140598.

80. National Institute for Health and Care Excellence. Microwave ablation for treating primary lung cancer and metastases in the lung (IPG469). London: National Institute for Health and Care Excellence; 2013. Available at: http://www.nice.org.uk/guidance/ipg469. Accessed October 6, 2015.

81. Vogl TJ, Naguib NN, Gruber-Rouh T, et al. Microwave ablation therapy: clinical utility in treatment of pulmonary metastases. Radiology 2011;261(2): 643–51.

82. Le QT, Loo BW, Ho A, et al. Results of a phase I dose-escalation study using single-fraction stereotactic radiotherapy for lung tumors. J Thorac Oncol 2006;1(8):802–9.

83. Yoon SM, Choi EK, Lee SW, et al. Clinical results of stereotactic body frame based fractionated radiation therapy for primary or metastatic thoracic tumors. Acta Oncol 2006;45(8):1108–14.

84. Hamamoto Y, Kataoka M, Yamashita M, et al. Local control of metastatic lung tumors treated with SBRT of 48 Gy in four fractions: in comparison with primary lung cancer. Jpn J Clin Oncol 2010;40(2): 125–9.

85. Yamamoto T, Jingu K, Shirata Y, et al. Outcomes after stereotactic body radiotherapy for lung tumors, with emphasis on comparison of primary lung cancer and metastatic lung tumors. BMC Cancer 2014;14:464.

86. Davis JN, Medbery C, Sharma S, et al. Stereotactic body radiotherapy for centrally located early-stage non-small cell lung cancer or lung metastases from the RSSearch((R)) patient registry. Radiat Oncol 2015;10(1):113.

87. Zhang Y, Xiao JP, Zhang HZ, et al. Stereotactic body radiation therapy favors long-term overall survival in patients with lung metastases: five-year experience of a single-institution. Chin Med J (Engl) 2011;124(24): 4132–7.

88. Ricardi U, Filippi AR, Guarneri A, et al. Stereotactic body radiation therapy for lung metastases. Lung Cancer 2012;75(1):77–81.

89. Inoue T, Oh RJ, Shiomi H, et al. Stereotactic body radiotherapy for pulmonary metastases. Prognostic factors and adverse respiratory events. Strahlenther Onkol 2013;189(4):285–92.

90. Osti MF, Carnevale A, Valeriani M, et al. Clinical outcomes of single dose stereotactic radiotherapy for lung metastases. Clin Lung Cancer 2013;14(6): 699–703.

91. Singh D, Chen Y, Hare MZ, et al. Local control rates with five-fraction stereotactic body radiotherapy for oligometastatic cancer to the lung. J Thorac Dis 2014;6(4):369–74.

92. Garcia-Cabezas S, Bueno C, Rivin E, et al. Lung metastases in oligometastatic patients: outcome with stereotactic body radiation therapy (SBRT). Clin Transl Oncol 2015;17(8):668–72.

93. Navarria P, Bueno C, Rivin E, et al. Stereotactic body radiation therapy for lung metastases from soft tissue sarcoma. Eur J Cancer 2015;51(5):668–74.

94. Nuyttens JJ, van der Voort van Zyp NC, Verhoef C, et al. Stereotactic body radiation therapy for oligometastases to the lung: a phase 2 study. Int J Radiat Oncol Biol Phys 2015;91(2):337–43.

95. Siva S, Kirby K, Caine H, et al. Comparison of single-fraction and multi-fraction stereotactic radiotherapy for patients with (18)F-fluorodeoxyglucose positron emission tomography-staged pulmonary oligometastases. Clin Oncol (R Coll Radiol) 2015;27(6):353–61.

96. Yan TD, King J, Sjarif A, et al. Percutaneous radiofrequency ablation of pulmonary metastases from colorectal carcinoma: prognostic determinants for survival. Ann Surg Oncol 2006;13(11):1529–37.

97. Simon CJ, Dupuy DE, DiPetrillo TA, et al. Pulmonary radiofrequency ablation: long-term safety and efficacy in 153 patients. Radiology 2007;243(1):268–75.

98. Petre EN, Jia X, Thornton RH, et al. Treatment of pulmonary colorectal metastases by radiofrequency ablation. Clin Colorectal Cancer 2013;12(1):37–44.

99. Koelblinger C, Strauss S, Gillams A. Outcome after radiofrequency ablation of sarcoma lung metastases. Cardiovasc Intervent Radiol 2014;37(1):147–53.

Lymphadenectomy During Pulmonary Metastasectomy

James Matthew Reinersman, MD[a],
Dennis A. Wigle, MD, PhD[b],*

KEYWORDS

• Lung metastasis • Metastasectomy • Lymphadenectomy

KEY POINTS

• Pulmonary metastasectomy improves survival in selected patients.
• The role of involvement of hilar and mediastinal lymph nodes remains poorly understood.
• This article summarizes the incidence and prognostic implications of thoracic lymph node metastases in the setting of pulmonary metastasectomy.

INTRODUCTION

The primary cause of death of patients with cancer is generally metastatic disease. Frequently, the lung is a site of metastatic disease and often portends widespread, systemic disease. The first pulmonary metastasectomy was reported in 1882.[1] Since this report, hundreds of articles have been published regarding the results of pulmonary metastasectomy. Despite a paucity of randomized clinical trial data, it is now generally accepted that overall survival for many tumor types is improved with resection of limited metastases in carefully selected patients.[2]

Despite improvements in disease-free and overall survival with pulmonary metastasectomy, few patients are effectively cured of their disease with this approach. Prognostic factors for patients undergoing pulmonary metastasectomy include cell type, time interval between primary tumor resection and identification of pulmonary metastases, number of pulmonary metastases, metastases to other sites, and the ability to completely resect all metastatic disease.

Only recently has there been significant attention given to the status and evaluation of lymph node metastases during pulmonary metastasectomy. Most surgical oncologists would agree that patients with bulky nodal metastases to the mediastinum are unlikely to benefit from surgical resection, and hence are not candidates for metastasectomy; this article analyzes only studies evaluating patients with minimal nodal disease burden or radiologically negative mediastinal nodes. This article focuses its discussion on the incidence of lymph node involvement, the impact on survival along with therapeutic implications, and recommendations regarding the management of these patients.

INCIDENCE

Pastorino and colleagues[2] validated the concept of pulmonary metastasectomy with the International Registry of Lung Metastasectomy published in 1997. Patients undergoing complete resection of all metastases were found to have an overall 5-year survival of 36% at 5 years, 26% at 10 years, and 22% at 15 years. However, the issue of mediastinal lymph node involvement by metastases was not addressed. The registry reported only a 5% incidence of lymph node metastases;

 a Division of Thoracic & Cardiovascular Surgery, Department of Surgery, University of Oklahoma Health Sciences Center, 920 Stanton L. Young Boulevard, WP 2230, Oklahoma City, OK 73104, USA; b Division of General Thoracic Surgery, Department of Surgery, Mayo Clinic, 200 First Street SW, Rochester, MN 55905, USA
* Corresponding author.
E-mail address: wigle.dennis@mayo.edu

Thorac Surg Clin 26 (2016) 35–40
http://dx.doi.org/10.1016/j.thorsurg.2015.09.005
1547-4127/16/$ – see front matter © 2016 Elsevier Inc. All rights reserved.

however, in this large database, only 4.6% of patients had lymph nodes resected or sampled. Therefore, this is not a representative statistical sample and likely largely underestimates the true incidence of lymph node metastases. Earlier reports suggested widely varying incidence of lymph node involvement for patients considered for pulmonary metastasectomy, ranging from 9.8% to 50%.[3,4] This wide variability is not unexpected given the time period, with chest radiograph being the main imaging modality available to identify a pulmonary metastasis.

In a Mayo Clinic pulmonary metastasectomy series, 70 patients had complete mediastinal lymphadenectomy with an incidence of lymph node metastases of 28.6% (20/70).[5] This included N1 level nodes in 9 patients (13%) N2 nodes in 8 patients (11%), and both in 3 patients (4%). A more recent Mayo Clinic report evaluated lymph node dissection in patients undergoing pulmonary metastasectomy for colorectal adenocarcinoma. From over 500 patients undergoing pulmonary metastasectomy, 319 patients underwent lymph node dissection, which revealed the incidence of positive lymph nodes to be 12.5% (40/319).[6]

Seebacher and colleagues[7] recently published their retrospective experience with lymph node evaluation in resections for pulmonary metastases. They found an incidence of 17% in all patients, with similar rates of involvement with radical lymphadenectomy 15.8% and sampling 18.8%. They found an incidence of 35.5% in patients with breast cancer (17 patients), 9.2% for colorectal cancer, and 20.8% in renal cell carcinoma.

Table 1 collates the list of the major papers to date illustrating the range of reported incidence of lymph node metastases at the time of pulmonary metastasectomy. The European Society of Thoracic Surgeons metastasectomy supplement combined 5 previous studies to come to a weighted average incidence of lymph node metastases of 22%.[8]

The role of thoracic lymph node dissection in pulmonary metastasectomy has been studied in a variety of patients with epithelial cancers, sarcomas, germ cell tumors, renal cancers, and melanoma. Some have argued that given sarcoma's low propensity for lymphatic metastases, the incidence of thoracic lymph node metastases with pulmonary metastasectomy should be low or nonexistent. This, however, has been refuted by multiple studies, and it is now known that sarcoma metastases to the lungs have a higher incidence of associated lymph node metastases than suspected. In Pfannschmidts's series of 70 patients with different types of sarcomas, 20.3% of patients (16 patients) had nodal metastases.[9]

In the same series, this was less than for colorectal (31.3%) and renal carcinomas (42.4%).

From the retrospective data available, it is clear that metastases to thoracic lymph nodes occur at a higher rate than previously recognized: roughly one in five patients. Several questions arise:

Does sampling versus lymphadenectomy make a difference?
What is the impact of these metastases on survival?
Do these patients still benefit from pulmonary metastasectomy?
What other therapeutic options are available?

Attempts to elicit potential risk factors for lymph node metastases have not been consistently reliable; however, this likely is related to study design and small patient numbers. Bolukbas and colleagues,[10] in their series of 165 patients, found that the number of pulmonary metastases has a nonlinear association with the risk of positive lymph node metastasis. The risk of lymph node metastasis increases 16% with each additional metastasis from 1 to 10; above 10 metastases the risk does not appear to increase further. Seebacher and colleagues also found the number of metastases to be prognostic for metastases to lymph nodes as well as metastasis size in their study of 209 patients with all types of cancers. A metastasis with a diameter of 2 cm or less had an incidence of lymph node involvement of 19.3%, but with a diameter of more than 4 cm, the incidence was 37.1% (P = .04). However, other authors have not found the number of metastases to be predictive of lymph node metastasis.[5,6]

LYMPH NODE SAMPLING VERSUS LYMPHADENECTOMY

Given the surprising incidence of lymph node metastases, a logical question is the appropriate surgical assessment of mediastinal lymph nodes at the time of metastasectomy. The following section will discuss what constitutes lymph node sampling versus dissection, and what data exist comparing the 2 methods.

The definition of a standard mediastinal lymph node sampling is considered as follows: right lung–lymph node stations 2R, 4R, 7, 9R, 10R; left lung–lymph node stations 5, 6, 7, 9L, and 10L. Lymphadenectomy for the right side includes removal of all lymph tissue in the 2R and 4R stations, defined by the takeoff of the right upper lobe bronchus, innominate artery, superior vena cava, and the trachea; removal of all tissue in the subcarinal space (station 7) as well as lymph nodes in the inferior pulmonary ligament and

Table 1
Incidence of lymph node involvement at time of pulmonary metastasectomy

Authors	Histology	Rate of Lymph Node Dissection	Sampling vs Lymphadenectomy	Incidence of Lymph Node Metastases
Seebacher et al,[7] 2015	Carcinomas and sarcomas	270/313 (86.3%)	Sampling 112, lymphadenectomy 158	46/270 (17%)
Renaud et al,[12] 2014	Renal cell	122/122 (100%)	Lymphadenectomy	43/122 (35%)
Bolukbas et al,[10] 2014	Colorectal	165/165 (100%)	Lymphadenectomy	37/165 (22.4%)
Renaud et al,[15] 2014	Colorectal	320/320 (100%)	Lymphadenectomy	140/320 (43.8%)
Hamaji et al,[6] 2012	Colorectal	319/518 (61.6%)	Lymphadenectomy	40/319 (12.5%)
Pfannschmidt et al,[9] 2006	Carcinomas & sarcomas	245/245 (100%)	Lymphadenectomy	80/245 (32.7%)
Murthy et al,[16] 2005	Renal cell	32/92 (34.8%)	Lymphadenectomy	12/32 (37.5%)
Ercan et al,[5] 2004	Carcinomas	107/883 (12.1%)	Lymphadenectomy	20/70 (28.6%)
Pfannschmidt et al,[17] 2003	Colorectal	167/167 (100%)	Lymphadenectomy	32/167 (19.1%)
Saito et al,[18] 2002	Colorectal	138/165 (83.6%)	Both	20/138 (14.5%)
Pfannschmidt et al,[19] 2002	Renal cell	191/191 (100%)	Lymphadenectomy	57/191 (29.8%)
Inoue et al,[20] 2000	Colorectal	25/25 (100%)	Sampling 17, lymphadenectomy 8	7/25 (28%)
Loehe et al,[21] 2001	Carcinomas & sarcomas	63/63 (100%)	Lymphadenectomy	9/63 (14.3%)
Kamiyoshihara et al,[14] 1998	Carcinomas	22/28 (78.6%)	Lymphadenectomy	6/22 (27.3%)
Pastorino et al,[2] 1997	Carcinomas & sarcomas	5%	Unknown	239/5206 (4.6%)
Okumura et al,[22] 1996	Colorectal	100/159 (62.9%)	Both	15/100 (15%)

Data from Refs.[2,5–7,9,10,15–22]

adjacent to the caudal half of the esophagus (stations 8 and 9). The left side includes the same dissection as the right for stations 7, 8, and 9, and also includes removing all tissue between the phrenic and vagus nerves extending down to the left main stem bronchus (stations 5 and 6).

Unfortunately, no clear comparative data exist assessing sampling versus lymphadenectomy during pulmonary metastasectomy. Most trials described in **Table 1** state that lymphadenectomy was performed as opposed to sampling. Some did include patients in both groups. However, few compared these techniques themselves. Seebacher and colleagues,[7] in a series of 270 procedures, performed lymphadenectomy in 158 procedures and sampling in 112, and found no difference in the incidence of lymph node metastases between the 2 groups. Furthermore, the 5-year survival (sampling 23.6%, lymphadenectomy 30.9%, $P = .29$) was not statistically different.

The only randomized data available assessing mediastinal lymphadenectomy versus sampling comes from the American College of Surgeons Oncology Group (ACOSOG) Z0030 Trial in primary nonsmall cell lung cancer (NSCLC). This trial was a randomized, multi-institutional, prospective study of lymphadenectomy versus sampling for patients with early stage NSCLC. No difference was found in local, regional, or distant recurrence in the 2 groups, and the 5-year disease-free survival was not different (69% for lymphadenectomy vs 68% for sampling; $P = .92$).[11]

The conclusion from Z0030 was that either procedure (lymph node sampling vs lymphadenectomy) was sufficient and necessary to adequately stage patients with clinical stage I NSCLC, with equivalent survival outcomes. Whether these data can be indirectly applied to pulmonary metastasectomy is an open question. Given the paucity of data, however, it would be reasonable to infer lymph node sampling as a minimal standard for mediastinal evaluation at the time of pulmonary metastasectomy.

PROGNOSIS

Given the current understanding of tumor biology, it is assumed that metastases to thoracic lymph nodes would convey a worse prognosis. However, no randomized controlled trials exist that compare outcomes with patients undergoing evaluation of thoracic lymph nodes at the time of metastasectomy. The retrospective data that do exist suggest a worse prognosis for patients with lymph node metastases across many different tumor types, summarized in **Table 2**.

Overall, if lymph nodes are not involved, 5-year survival ranges from 24.7% to 50%. This compares to patients with metastatically involved lymph nodes having a 0% to 24% 5-year survival. Not every series available in the literature finds that lymph node metastases predict a worse survival; however, some studies are difficult to interpret given the degree of lymph node sampling or the small number of patients involved. Most of the key studies with larger populations have been for patients with metastatic colorectal cancer; however, a few evaluate other cancers also. An overall review of the current data does support the conclusion that metastases to thoracic lymph nodes portend a worse overall survival.

In the series by Ercan and colleagues,[5] which expressly evaluated the prognosis of lymph node metastasis, lymph node metastases were found to adversely affect survival, with 3-year survival of 69% without lymph node metastases versus 38% for those with metastases. N1 versus N2 positivity did not appear to confer a difference in survival. Only 2 patients survived to 5 years, and both of these were patients with renal cell carcinoma. Hamaji and colleagues[6] more recently asked the question whether lymph node dissection is required in metastasectomy for colorectal cancer. They found that the only significant prognostic factor for survival after pulmonary metastasectomy was mediastinal lymph node metastasis. Patients who underwent no lymph node dissection and those with negative lymph node dissections had 5-year survival rates of 48.3% and 49.3%, and 10-year survival rates of 29.4% and 27.5%, compared to those with a positive lymph node dissection having both 5- and 10 year survival rates of approximately 21%.

Renaud and authors similarly found in an analysis of 122 patients with renal cell carcinoma metastases that lymph node involvement did have an adverse effect on survival. 107 months if there was no lymph node involvement versus 37 months with lymph node involvement.[12]

Pfannschmidt and colleagues[9] showed that median survival was also worse with involved lymph nodes. Median survival was 63.9 months if N0 disease, 32.7 months with N1 disease, and following complete resection 32.7 months for patients with N1 disease versus 20.6 months for patients with N1 and N2 disease. However, Hamaji and colleagues[6] found no difference in survival based on N station status (32.5 months for N1 level vs 34 months for N2 level, $P = .69$) or between single-station and multistation metastasis (35.5 months for single vs 30 months for multiple stations, $P = .78$). Renaud and colleagues[12] similarly found no survival difference in N1 versus N2 lymph node involvement in patients with renal cell carcinoma.

Table 2
Survival with lymph node involvement at the time of pulmonary metastasectomy

Authors	Histology	5 y Survival		
		Negative Nodes	Positive Nodes	P value
Seebacher et al,[7] 2015	Carcinomas & sarcomas	30.20%	25%	P = .1
Renaud et al,[12] 2014	Renal cell	71%	37%	P = .003
Bolukbas et al,[10] 2014	Colorectal	59.00%	23%	P = .03
Hamaji et al,[6] 2012	Colorectal	49.30%	20.70%	P = .047
Ercan et al,[5] 2004	Carcinomas	68% (3 y)	38% (3 y)	P<.001
Pfannschmidt et al,[17] 2003	Colorectal	38.70%	0%	P<.03
Kamiyoshihara et al,[14] 1998	Carcinomas	24.70%	0%	NS
Pfannschmidt et al,[19] 2002	Renal cell	42%	24%	P = .016
Inoue et al,[20] 2000	Colorectal	49.50%	14.30%	P = .003
Saito et al,[18] 2002	Colorectal	48.5% (4 y)	6.2% (4 y)	P<.001
Okumura et al,[22] 1996	Colorectal	50%	6.70%	P = .0004
Piltz et al,[23] 2002	Renal cell	48%	0%	P<.001

Data from Refs.[5–7,10,12,17–20,22,23]

THERAPEUTIC IMPLICATIONS

Given this difference in survival based on thoracic lymph node involvement, some authors have argued for more thorough preoperative evaluation of patients prior to pulmonary metastasectomy.[8] Menon and colleagues[13] reported using videome-diastinoscopy preoperatively prior to metastasectomy for assessment of mediastinal lymph nodes. The European Society of Thoracic Surgeons supplement in the Journal of Thoracic Oncology in 2010, discussing thoracic lymph node involvement with pulmonary metastasectomy, made a number of controversial conclusions in this area. They argued that best practice would be to perform mediastinoscopy prior to metastasectomy, and to exclude patients with thoracic nodal involvement from pulmonary metastasectomy.[8]

Despite acknowledging a worse prognosis with lymph node metastases, the authors would argue that excluding patients with nodal disease from pulmonary metastasectomy may be unwarranted. Although any potential therapeutic effect of thoracic mediastinal lymph node dissection is unclear, a thorough pathologic assessment of hilar and mediastinal lymph nodes is necessary at the time of metastasectomy to adequately assess disease burden given the impact on prognosis. Hamaji noted a worse survival with lymph node positivity, but did note 3 long-term survivors (>5 years) in their group of patients with a positive lymphadenectomy.[6] One of these 3 patients had multiple positive lymph node stations. Kamiyoshihara and colleagues[14] argue that a systematic and radical mediastinal dissection can be curative, although this remains controversial. Prevailing opinion suggests the strongest role for lymph node assessment to be that of evaluating disease status and burden.

Although many of these issues will remain controversial, the authors believe the primary benefit of lymph node assessment during pulmonary metastasectomy is to allow for stratification of a patient into potential treatment strategies. For example, patients with completely resected disease and no positive thoracic lymph nodes may be safely observed, as opposed to patients with thoracic lymph node involvement who may be candidates for further systemic therapy. Clearly, this is an area where consensus statements are unlikely to keep pace with the development of novel therapeutics, and histology-specific approaches are likely to evolve. In the setting of metastatic disease, the role of local therapies such as surgery will only expand with the development of more effective systemic treatments. This is particularly relevant in the current era of ever-changing targeted therapeutics, and the recent exciting development of successful immunotherapies.

SUMMARY

Pulmonary metastasectomy continues to be an effective approach to prolong survival in appropriately selected patients. In regards to lymph node status at the time of metastasectomy, the authors draw the following conclusions:

1. The incidence of lymphatic spread is more common than previously recognized, with an

estimate of 20% to 25% across multiple tumor types. The authors would recommend all patients undergoing pulmonary metastasectomy to have a concomitant lymph node sampling or dissection for assessment of disease burden.

2. The presence of metastatically involved lymph nodes adversely affects survival. What remains unclear is whether N1 vs N2, or the number of stations involved affects survival differently.

3. The authors recommend patients with lymph node metastases, if discovered preoperatively, still be offered metastasectomy selectively, since survival has been demonstrated in a limited number of select cases. The role of surgery for pulmonary metastasectomy in the patient with nodal metastases will likely expand with ongoing improvements in targeted and immunotherapies.

REFERENCES

1. Weinlechner J. Tumoren an der Brust und deren Behandlung Resektion der Rippen, Eroeffnug der Brusthuoehle, partielle Entfernung der Lunge. Wien Med Wochenschr 1882;20–1 [in German].

2. Pastorino U, Buyse M, Friedel G, et al. Long-term results of lung metastasectomy: prognostic analyses based on 5206 cases. J Thorac Cardiovasc Surg 1997;113:37–49.

3. Thomford NR, Woolner LB, Clagett T. The surgical treatment of metastatic tumors in the lung. J Thorac Cardiovasc Surg 1965;49:357–63.

4. Cahan WG, Gastro EB, Hajdu SI. Therapeutic pulmonary resection of colonic carcinoma metastatic to lung. Dis Colon Rectum 1974;17:302–9.

5. Ercan S, Nichols FC, Trastek VF, et al. Prognostic significance of lymph node metastasis found during pulmonary metastasectomy for extrapulmonary carcinoma. Ann Thorac Surg 2004;77:1786–91.

6. Hamaji M, Cassivi SD, Shen KR, et al. Is lymph node dissection required in pulmonary metastasectomy for colorectal adenocarcinoma? Ann Thorac Surg 2012;94:1796–801.

7. Seebacher G, Decker S, Fischer JR, et al. Unexpected lymph node disease in resections for pulmonary metastases. Ann Thorac Surg 2015;99:231–7.

8. Garcia-Yuste M, Cassivi S, Paleru C. Thoracic lymphatic involvement in patients having pulmonary metastasectomy. J Thorac Oncol 2010;5:S166–9.

9. Pfannschmidt J, Klode J, Muley T, et al. Nodal involvement at the time of pulmonary metastasectomy: experience in 245 patients. Ann Thorac Surg 2006;81:448–54.

10. Bolukbas S, Sponholz S, Kudelin N, et al. Risk factors for lymph node metastases and

11. Darling GE, Allen MS, Decker PA, et al. Randomized trial of mediastinal lymph node sampling versus complete lymphadenectomy during pulmonary resection in the patient with N0 or N1 (less than hilar) non-small cell carcinoma: results of the American College of Surgery Oncology Group Z0030 Trial. J Thorac Cardiovasc Surg 2011;141:662–70.

12. Renaud S, Falcoz PE, Alifano M, et al. Systematic lymph node dissection in lung metastasectomy of renal cell carcinoma: an 18 years of experience. J Surg Oncol 2014;109:823–9.

13. Menon A, Milton R, Thorpe JA, et al. The value of video-assisted mediastinoscopy in pulmonary metastasectomy. Eur J Cardiothorac Surg 2007;32:351–4.

14. Kamiyoshihara M, Hirai T, Kawashima O, et al. The surgical treatment of metastatic tumors in the lung: is lobectomy with mediastinal lymph node dissection suitable treatment? Oncol Rep 1998;5:453–7.

15. Renaud S, Alifano M, Falcoz PE, et al. Does nodal status influence survival? Results of a 19-year lymphadenectomy experience during lung metastasectomy of colorectal cancer. Interact Cardiovasc Thorac Surg 2014;18:482–7.

16. Murthy SC, Kwhanmien K, Rice TW, et al. Can we predict long-term survival after pulmonary metastasectomy for renal cell carcinoma? Ann Thorac Surg 2005;79:996–1003.

17. Pfannschmidt J, Muley T, Hoffman H, et al. Prognostic factors and survival after complete resection of pulmonary metastases from colorectal carcinoma: experience in 167 patients. J Thorac Cardiovasc Surg 2003;126:732–9.

18. Saito Y, Omiya H, Kohno K, et al. Pulmonary metastasectomy for 165 patients with colorectal carcinoma: a prognostic assessment. J Thorac Cardiovasc Surg 2002;124:1007–13.

19. Pfannschmidt J, Hoffman H, Muley T, et al. Prognostic factors for survival after pulmonary resection of metastatic renal cell carcinoma. Ann Thorac Surg 2002;74:1653–7.

20. Inoue M, Kotake Y, Nakagawa K, et al. Surgery for pulmonary metastases from colorectal carcinoma. Ann Thorac Surg 2000;70:380–3.

21. Loehe F, Kobinger S, Hatz RA, et al. Value of systematic mediastinal lymph node dissection during pulmonary metastasectomy. Ann Thorac Surg 2001;72:225–9.

22. Okumura S, Kondo H, Tsuboi M, et al. Pulmonary resection for metastatic colorectal cancer: experiences with 159 patients. J Thorac Cardiovasc Surg 1996;112:867–74.

23. Piltz S, Meimarakis G, Wichmann MW, et al. Long-term results after pulmonary resection of renal cell carcinoma metastases. Ann Thorac Surg 2002;73:1082–7.

Results of Pulmonary Resection
Colorectal Carcinoma

Karen J. Dickinson, MBBS, BSc, MD, FRCS,
Shanda H. Blackmon, MD, MPH*

KEYWORDS

- Colorectal cancer • Metastasis • Metastasectomy • Pulmonary resection

KEY POINTS

- Five year survival in patients undergoing pulmonary metastasectomy for colorectal cancer has been reported to exceed 50% in some studies.
- Care should be taken when interpreting survival data, as there are few randomized controlled trials and reported series include a highly selected group of patients.
- Factors that may predict improved survival after pulmonary metastasectomy include fewer nodules, longer disease-free interval, and absence of lymph node involvement.
- New studies indicate that a lymphadenectomy should accompany metastasectomy.
- Patients should be carefully selected for metastasectomy based on stability of disease (no increase in number of nodules and no increase in size of nodules over sequential scans), ability to tolerate resection, and controlled extrathoracic disease.

INTRODUCTION

The management of colorectal lung metastases is an important clinical problem. Colorectal cancer is one of the commonest tumors diagnosed in the West.[1] In 10% to 20% of patients the disease is metastatic at the time of presentation.[2] For patients with stage IV disease who are untreated, the median survival is 5 to 6 months.[2] In these patients, the conventional treatment with chemotherapy regimens based on 5-fluorouracil results in a 5-year survival of approximately 5%. Any intervention that could prolong quality of life in patients with metastatic disease is important.

Current management of metastatic colorectal cancer includes pulmonary and hepatic metastasectomy in selected patients, usually in conjunction with chemotherapy. Five-year survival rates of up to 54% have been reported in selected patients undergoing pulmonary metastasectomy,

although this is not based on randomized clinical trials.[3] The benefits of pulmonary metastasectomy in colorectal cancer are controversial, given the paucity of data on survival in comparable patients not undergoing lung resection. Despite this, the surgical approach to pulmonary metastasectomy has developed significantly since an early description by Blalock[4] of pneumonectomy to manage metastatic disease. The focus in thoracic surgical practice has shifted toward exploring the option of lung preservation, whether pulmonary metastasectomies or primary lung cancers are being treated.[5] Although several controversies exist and divide the opinion of thoracic surgeons with regard to the management of colorectal lung metastases,[6] 92% perform nonanatomic parenchyma-preserving wedge resections for these cases.[7] Preservation of lung parenchyma in these patients allows repeated surgical resections and may therefore prolong their survival.

Disclosure for financial support: no disclosures.
Division of General Thoracic Surgery, Mayo Clinic, 200 First Street Southwest, Rochester, MN 55905, USA
* Corresponding author.
E-mail address: Blackmon.shanda@mayo.edu

Thorac Surg Clin 26 (2016) 41–47
http://dx.doi.org/10.1016/j.thorsurg.2015.09.006
1547-4127/16/$ – see front matter © 2016 Elsevier Inc. All rights reserved.

The clinical evidence for the management of these patients is evolving, as are the technologies available to thoracic surgeons with which to treat them. This article highlights the areas of controversy and current evidence with reference to the outcomes of patients undergoing pulmonary metastasectomy for colorectal carcinoma metastases. Also discussed are emerging technologies and future directions for managing these patients.

PATIENT SELECTION AND OPERATIVE TECHNIQUE

For a patient to be considered for pulmonary metastasectomy, the disease within the chest should be stable on sequential imaging, the primary disease should be controlled or controllable, and the metastases anatomically suitable for resection. The patient should be able to tolerate the anesthesia and the proposed lung resection. The aim of pulmonary metastasectomy is to resect the metastatic lesions with negative margins (R0). Anatomic resection of pulmonary metastases does not confer superior survival when compared with wedge resection.[8] A lymphadenectomy should also be performed. Preservation of lung parenchyma is important to maximize lung function and allow further resection if necessary. Pulmonary metastases are often located at the periphery of the lung, making them amenable to wedge resection. Lobectomy or even pneumonectomy is less commonly performed. A pneumonectomy should never be performed when the diagnosis of the mass is unknown. When an anatomic resection is required, the authors suggest that segmentectomy should be preferred over lobectomy. The International Registry of Lung Metastases reported that 20% of patients underwent multiple resections.[9] Despite this, studies report rates of less than 10% for segmentectomies to treat colorectal metastases.[10,11] Another consideration for these patients, 1 in 5 of whom will be undergoing multiple resections, is the use of a minimally invasive approach (video-assisted thoracoscopic surgery [VATS]). This approach is associated with less postoperative pain and intrathoracic adhesion formation.[12,13]

A criticism of VATS is that the entire lung cannot be palpated as readily as via a thoracotomy. Missed metastases have been reported to occur in up to 56% of patients.[14,15] In fact, 65% of thoracic surgeons believe that palpation of the lung is required for adequate identification of lung nodules.[7] Even so, missed metastases do not seem to affect patient survival.[12,16] In the context of careful postoperative surveillance for

these patients, improved localization of nodules, enhanced skill of surgeons performing VATS wedge resection, ablation, segmentectomy, or, where indicated, lobectomy can be associated with fewer complications and shorter hospital stay.[17] In the authors' experience, conversion to open surgery is rare. Such conversion is associated with inadequate visualization of hilar structures or relevant anatomy, in addition to bleeding.

Newer approaches to the resection of pulmonary colorectal metastases are aimed at reducing the morbidity of the resection. These techniques include pulmonary metastasectomy via a single-incision subxiphoid approach.[18] This method allows both lungs to be accessed in one position and via one incision, and provides exciting opportunities for development of less invasive and arguably less morbid procedures to deal with pulmonary metastases. Other techniques under investigation include isolated lung perfusion with various chemotherapeutic agents in patients with unresectable lung metastases.[19]

NONOPERATIVE AND HYBRID TREATMENT OF PULMONARY METASTASES

In keeping with the parenchyma-sparing approach, there are several nonoperative strategies that can be used alone or in combination with surgical resection, including radiofrequency ablation (RFA), cryoablation (CA), and microwave ablation (MWA). RFA causes focal coagulation of tissue and subsequent necrosis. This treatment is particularly suitable for small lesions, and progression can occur in up to 10% of patients after RFA treatment. RFA has important benefits including preservation of lung function, repeatability, and the ability to be combined with other treatments, including surgical resection. The combination of RFA and surgery may allow more lung parenchyma to be preserved. RFA alone is associated with 45% to 55% survival at 5 years, although in only a highly selected group of patients.[20] RFA can be considered for the treatment of patients for whom surgical resection is not possible because of comorbid conditions.[21] More recently, the outcomes of surgery and RFA in combination as a hybrid approach are being investigated. This strategy may allow treatment of anatomically unresectable tumors in combination with those amenable for wedge resection. The use of RFA and subsequent resection of these tumors also allows the study of the effects of the treatment on the metastatic tumor and prognostic indicators to be identified, such as those that predict which patients will do well with surgical metastasectomy. Stereotactic body radiotherapy is another parenchyma-preserving treatment that can be used alone or in conjunction with surgical resection to treat pulmonary metastases.[22] The authors' institution is currently studying the efficacy of CA and MWA for pulmonary metastases.

PROGNOSTIC FACTORS FOR COLORECTAL PULMONARY METASTASECTOMY

The main criticism of the literature pertaining to pulmonary metastasectomy in colorectal cancer is that it consists largely of retrospective reviews of single-center experiences. There are several systematic reviews analyzing the current evidence, although there is significant heterogeneity between the studies.[3,23–25] This divergence is related not only to variations in surgical practice but also to differences in data collection between studies. Five-year survival in these studies is recorded as being up to 54%. The main criticism is that there is no published comparison of survival data in those patients selected for metastasectomy had they not undergone surgery. It may be that these patients would have done well with or without surgical intervention, and that their favorable clinical/pathologic status made them good surgical candidates. Although not a direct comparison of patients undergoing or not undergoing metastasectomy, the FACS randomized controlled trial assessed the effect of earlier detection of metastatic colorectal cancer on increasing the rate of pulmonary metastastectomy.[26] This trial did not demonstrate an effect on the survival of these patients.

These observations have led to the recruitment of patients to the PulMiCC trial, a randomized controlled trial assessing the effect on survival of pulmonary metastasectomy. To date more than 300 patients have entered stage I and 80 patients have entered stage II of the trial.[27]

Despite weaknesses in the literature, information with regard to factors that may be predictive of outcome in these patients has been obtained. Determining patients 'prognostic scores' based on preoperative and perioperative criteria is helpful not only in selecting patients who will do well with metastasectomy but also in counseling them appropriately.

Prognostic factors that have been suggested include the size of metastasis, the nodal status, the distribution of metastatic disease, and the preoperative carcinoembryonic antigen (CEA) levels. The disease-free interval may also be associated with patient prognosis (**Table 1**). Other tumor markers (eg, EGFR, BRAF, KRAS, HSP-27) are not in routine clinical use for risk assessment, but recent evidence suggests their prognostic importance.[28]

Table 1
Summary of survival outcomes and prognostic factors in recently published studies

	Patients (N)	5-y Survival (%)	Prognostic Factor
Zink et al,[45] 2001	110	32.6	Number of mets, CEA, size of mets
Rena et al,[46] 2002	80	41.1	DFI, number of mets, CEA
Saito et al,[47] 2002	165	39.6	LN mets, CEA
Pfannschmidt et al,[48] 2003	167	32.4	LN mets, CEA, number of mets
Inoue et al,[49] 2000	128	45.3	Primary tumor stage, distribution of mets
Melloni et al,[50] 2006	81	42.0	Primary tumor stage, complete resection
Yedibela et al,[51] 2006	153	37.0	Number of mets, DFI, transfusion
Welter et al,[52] 2007	169	39.1	DFI, number of mets, LN mets
Lin et al,[53] 2009	63	43.9	DFI, type of resection
Onaitis et al,[54] 2009	378	78.0[a]	Age, sex, DFI, number of mets
Watanabe et al,[55] 2009	113	67.8	CEA, lymphatic invasion
Landes et al,[56] 2010	40	43.4	Prior history of liver mets
Riquet et al,[57] 2010	127	41.0	Complete resection
Zabaleta et al,[58] 2011	84	54.0	Prior history of liver mets, LN mets, DFI, number of mets

Abbreviations: CEA, carcinoembryonic antigen; DFI, disease-free interval; LN, lymph node; mets, metastasis.
[a] Indicates 3-year survival rate.

SIZE AND LOCATION OF METASTASIS

The size of the metastasis is important, as this may affect the resectability, but more crucial is the location in relation to hilar structures and segmental anatomy. Some studies have shown that size is associated with poorer prognosis.[29–31] There is conflicting evidence with regard to the location of metastasis and survival. It has been recorded that unilateral location is associated with better survival,[32] although other studies have shown no difference in survival in those patients with bilateral metastasectomy.[33]

NUMBER OF METASTASES

There are no current recommendations for the maximum number of colorectal pulmonary metastases above which one should not resect. This decision is made on an individual basis and is determined by the comorbidities of the patient, the status of the primary tumor, the resectability of other extrapulmonary metastases, and the anatomic location of the pulmonary metastases. It has been shown that a greater number of lung metastases predict poorer survival after resection of pulmonary colorectal cancer metastases. The number of lung metastases present was able to predict the risk of recurrence in the lung. More than 3 metastases at resection were associated with poorer survival (hazard ratio [HR], 1.15; 95% confidence interval [CI], 1.024–1.282; $P = .018$), and more than 3 metastasis present at first metastasectomy predicted recurrence of disease in the lung (HR, 1.19; 95% CI, 1.071–1.321; $P = .001$).[34] Other studies have also demonstrated a relationship between number of pulmonary metastases and survival,[35–37] and have reported no difference in survival between patients who underwent metastasectomy for solitary compared with multiple lesions, although this may be in relation to the preoperative and intraoperative identification of "occult" metastases or micrometastases.[38,39]

LYMPH NODE METASTASES

Gonzales and colleagues,[25] in their meta-analysis, have shown that hilar and mediastinal lymph node involvement was associated with poor patient outcome. The recommendations of this group were that thorough nodal staging should be performed before resection in patients being considered for pulmonary metastasectomy for colorectal cancer (ie, PET/computed tomography). Moreover, they suggest that mediastinoscopy should be performed in these patients when there is any suspicion of nodal involvement. More recently, Renaud and colleagues[40] have demonstrated that patients with N0 disease had a median survival of 94 months compared with 42 months for those with N+ disease (p<0.001, odds ratio = 0.573 [0.329–1], p=0.05).

In light of these data, a survey of current practice performed by the European Society of Thoracic Surgeons has shown that, while 65% of surgeons who responded would consider pathologically positive nodes a contraindication to pulmonary metastasectomy, a similar proportion never or rarely perform mediastinoscopy before their metastasectomies. One-third of the thoracic surgeons surveyed did not perform any sort of nodal dissection.[7]

PREOPERATIVE CARCINOEMBRYONIC ANTIGEN LEVEL

In the surveillance of colorectal cancer, CEA is important in alerting the clinician to the possibility of disease recurrence or metastasis. On the apical surface of the epithelial cells of the colon. There is conflicting evidence as to whether preoperative CEA is associated with poor outcome after pulmonary metastasectomy. Increased CEA has been associated with poor survival,[39] although one study has shown that, in patients undergoing pulmonary metastasectomy with a CEA level of at least 5 ng/mL, survival was 53%.[41] There is no doubt that postmetastasectomy monitoring of CEA is essential for the detection of disease recurrence.

DISEASE-FREE INTERVAL

Systematic review of the published literature has not suggested that an increased disease-free interval is associated with survival benefit.[23] Only 6 studies in the review by Pfannschmidt and colleagues[23] demonstrated that a short disease-free interval is associated with poorer prognosis. Despite this, it is reasonable to suggest that these patients, and those with metastasis at the time of diagnosis of the primary tumor, may have a more aggressive tumor biology and, therefore, poorer survival. It has been suggested that a disease-free interval of less than 1 year is associated with poorer survival,[10] and in the absence of more robust data this should be considered when assessing patients for pulmonary metastasectomy.

Current data with regard to the benefits of pulmonary metastasectomy for colorectal cancer are flawed. However, prognostic factors have been identified that may be associated with increased risk of recurrence and reduced survival. When managing these patients, the "prognostic score" should be analyzed and accounted for when the decision to resect these metastases is made.

NEW PROGNOSTIC INDICATORS

Several recent studies are investigating novel markers in colorectal pulmonary metastases. These markers may be useful as prognostic indicators and to predict patient survival after future study. Schweiger and colleagues[42] have demonstrated that patients with KRAS mutations were at higher risk of early pulmonary recurrence and also had a more diffuse pattern of metastatic disease. When patients with mutant KRAS (mKRAS) and mutant BRAF (mBRAF) were studied alongside those with wild-type KRAS and BRAF, 5-year overall survival was 0% for patients with mBRAF, 44% for patients with mKRAS, and 100% for wild-type patients.[43] Further study has been directed at heat-shock protein (Hsp27) in patients with colorectal cancer undergoing pulmonary metastasectomy. Hsp27 is a protein that is upregulated on activated fibroblasts during wound healing and is elevated in various disease states, including cancer. Cancer-associated fibroblasts (CAF) are important as prognostic and predictive markers in malignancies. Schweiger and colleagues[44] measured the levels of Hsp27 produced by CAF in patients with colorectal cancer and pulmonary metastasectomy. Strong expression of Hsp27 was associated with decreased recurrence-free survival in these patients. Typing patients in this manner could allow for assessment of a prognostic score to direct surgical treatment and allow appropriate counseling of the patient.

THE FUTURE

The future of colorectal metastasectomy will include a combination of minimally invasive approaches, lung parenchyma-sparing technology, and likely combinations of ablation and surgery used in conjunction with novel chemotherapeutics and targeted therapy. As ablative techniques improve, they will certainly be highly utilized to save lung when lesions would have otherwise required a lobectomy or a large parenchymal resection for removal of disease. The authors' center routinely conducts a lung ablation tumor board that reviews lesions and patients to develop a strategy for disease removal while sparing healthy lung tissue. This team comprises radiologists, interventional radiologists, thoracic surgeons, oncologists, radiation oncologists, and pulmonologists, who strategize to develop a patient-centered care plan. This multidisciplinary approach to the management of colorectal pulmonary metastases is essential for successful patient outcomes.

REFERENCES

1. Jemal A, Bray F, Canter MM, et al. Global cancer statistics. CA Cancer J Clin 2011;61:69–90.
2. Labianca R, Beretta GD, Kildani B, et al. Colon cancer. Crit Rev Oncol Hematol 2010;74:106–33.
3. Fiorentino F, Hunt I, Teoh K, et al. Pulmonary metastasectomy in colorectal cancer: a systematic review and quantitative synthesis. J R Soc Med 2010;103:60–6.
4. Blalock A. Recent advances in surgery. N Engl J Med 1944;231:261–7.
5. Villamizar N, Swanson S. Lobectomy vs. segmentectomy for NSCLC (T<2cm). Ann Cardiothorac Surg 2014;3:160–6.
6. Fiorentino F, Treasure T. Pulmonary metastasectomy for colorectal carcinoma: making the case for a randomized controlled trial in the zone of uncertainty. J Thorac Cardiovasc Surg 2013;145: 748–52.
7. Internullo E, Cassivi SD, Van Raemdonck D, et al. Pulmonary metastasectomy: a survey of current practice amongst members of the European Society of Thoracic Surgeons. J Thorac Oncol 2008;3: 1257–66.
8. Lo Faso F, Salaini L, Lembo R, et al. Thoracoscopic lung metastasectomies: a 10-year single center experience. Surg Endosc 2013;27:1938–44.
9. Pastorino U, Buyse M, Friedel G, et al, The International Registry of Lung. Long-term results of lung metastasectomy: prognostic analysis based on 5206 cases. J Thorac Cardiovasc Surg 1997;113:37–49.
10. Onaitis MW, Petersen RP, Haney JC, et al. Prognostic factors for recurrence after pulmonary resection of colorectal cancer metastases. Ann Thorac Surg 2009;87:1684–8.
11. Rena O, Casadio C, Viano F, et al. Pulmonary resection for metastases from colorectal cancer: factors influencing prognosis. Twenty-year experience. Eur J Cardiothorac Surg 2002;21:906–12.
12. Mutsaerts El, Zoetmulder FA, Meijer S, et al. Long-term survival of thoracoscopic metastasectomy vs metastasectomy by thoracotomy in patients with a solitary pulmonary lesion. Eur J Surg Oncol 2002; 28:864–8.
13. Gossot D, Radu C, Girard P. Resection of pulmonary metastases from sarcoma: can patients benefit from a less invasive approach? Ann Thorac Surg 2009; 87:238–43.
14. Mutsaerts El, Zoetmulder FA, Meijer S, et al. Outcome of thoracoscopic pulmonary metastasectomy

evaluated by confirmatory thoracotomy. Ann Thorac Surg 2001;72:230–3.

15. McCormack PM, Bains MS, Begg CB, et al. Role of video assisted thoracoscopic surgery in the treatment of pulmonary metastases: results of a prospective trial. Ann Thorac Surg 1996;62: 213–6.

16. Nakas A, Klimatsidas MN, Entwistle J, et al. Video-assisted versus open pulmonary metastasectomy: the surgeon's finger or the radiologist's eye? Eur J Cardiothorac Surg 2009;36:469–74.

17. Leshnower BG, Miller DL, Fernandes FG, et al. Video assisted thoracoscopic surgery segmentectomy: a safe and effective procedure. Ann Thorac Surg 2010;89:1571–6.

18. Surda T, Ahikari S, Tochii S, et al. Single incision subxiphoid approach for bilateral metastasectomy. Ann Thorac Surg 2014;97:718–9.

19. Den Hengst WA, Hendriks JM, Balduyck B, et al. Phase II multicenter clinical trial of pulmonary metastasectomy and isolated lung perfusion with melphalan in patients with resectable lung metastases. J Thorac Oncol 2014;9:1547–53.

20. Hiraki T, Gobara H, Iguchi T, et al. Radiofrequency ablation as treatment for pulmonary metastasis of colorectal cancer. World J Gastroenterol 2014;20: 988–96.

21. Chua TC, Sarkar A, Saxena A, et al. Long-term outcome of image guided percutaneous radiofrequency ablation of lung metastases: an open labeled prospective trial of 148 patients. Ann Oncol 2010;21:2017–22.

22. Carvajal C, Navarro-Martin A, Cacicedo J, et al. Stereotactic body radiotherapy for colorectal lung oligometastases: preliminary single-institution results. J BUON 2015;20:158–65.

23. Pfannschmidt J, Dienemann H, Hoffmann H. Surgical resection of pulmonary metastasis from colorectal cancer: a systematic review of published series. Ann Thorac Surg 2007;84: 324–38.

24. Salah S, Watanabe K, Welter S, et al. Colorectal cancer pulmonary oligometastases: pooled analysis and construction of a clinical lung metastasectomy project model. Ann Oncol 2012;23: 2649–55.

25. Gonzalez M, Ponet A, Combescure C, et al. Risk factors for survival after lung metastasectomy in colorectal cancer patients: a systematic review and meta-analysis. Ann Surg Oncol 2013;20: 572–9.

26. Primrose JN, Perera R, Gray A, et al. Effect of 3 to 5 years of scheduled CEA and CT follow up to detect recurrence of colorectal cancer: the FACS randomized clinical trial. JAMA 2014;311:263–70.

27. Migliore M, Milosevic M, Lees B, et al. Finding the evidence for pulmonary metastasectomy in colorectal cancer: the PulMiCC trial. Future Oncol 2015;11:15–8.

28. Kim HK, Cho JH, Lee HY, et al. Pulmonary metastasectomy for colorectal cancer: how many nodules, how many times? World J Gastroenterol 2014;20: 6133–45.

29. Vogelsang H, Haas S, Hierholser C, et al. Factors influencing survival after resection of pulmonary metastases from colorectal cancer. Br J Surg 2004;91: 1066–71.

30. Brasa T, Suzuki K, Yoshida S, et al. Prediction of prognosis and surgical indicators for pulmonary metastasectomy from colorectal cancer. Ann Thorac Surg 2006;82:254–60.

31. Javed MA, Sheel AR, Sheikh AA, et al. Size of metastatic deposit affects prognosis in patients undergoing pulmonary metastasectomy for colorectal cancer. Ann R Coll Surg Engl 2014; 96:32–6.

32. Inoue I, Ohta M, Iuchi K, et al. Benefits of surgery for patients with pulmonary metastases from colorectal carcinoma. Ann Thorac Surg 2004;78: 238–44.

33. Riquet M, Foucault C, Cazes A, et al. Pulmonary resection for metastases of colorectal adenocarcinoma. Ann Thorac Surg 2010;89:375–80.

34. Blackmon SH, Stephens EH, Correa AM, et al. Predictors of recurrent pulmonary metastases and survival after pulmonary metastasectomy for colorectal cancer. Ann Thorac Surg 2012;94: 1802–9.

35. McAfee MK, Allen MS, Trastek VF, et al. Pulmonary resection for metastases from colorectal cancer. Chest 2001;119:1069–72.

36. Okumura S, Kondo H, Tsuboi M, et al. Pulmonary resection for metastatic colorectal cancer: experience with 159 patients. J Thorac Cardiovasc Surg 1996;112:867–74.

37. Girard P, Ducreux M, Baldeyrou P, et al. Surgery for lung metastasis from colorectal cancer: analysis of prognostic factors. J Clin Oncol 1996;14: 2047–53.

38. Inoue M, Kotake Y, Nakagawa K, et al. Surgery for pulmonary metastases from colorectal carcinoma. Ann Thorac Surg 2000;70:380–3.

39. Sakamoto T, Tsubota N, Iwanaga K, et al. Pulmonary resection for metastases from colorectal cancer. Chest 2001;119:1069–72.

40. Renaud S, Alifano M, Falcoz PE, et al. Does nodal status influence survival? Results of a 19-year systematic lymphadenectomy experience during lung metastasectomy of colorectal cancer. Interact Cardiovasc Thorac Surg 2014;18:482–7.

41. Watanabe K, Nagai K, Kobayashi A, et al. Factors influencing survival after complete resection of pulmonary metastases from colorectal cancer. Br J Surg 2009;96:1058–65.

42. Schweiger T, Hegedus B, Mikolowsky C, et al. EGFR, BRAF and KRAS status in patients undergoing pulmonary metastasectomy from primary colorectal carcinoma: a prospective follow-up study. Ann Surg Oncol 2014;21:946–54.

43. Renaud S, Romain B, Falcoz PE, et al. KRAS and BRAF mutations are prognostic biomarkers in patients undergoing lung metastasectomy of colorectal cancer. Br J Cancer 2015;112:720–8.

44. Schweiger T, Nikolowsky C, Starlinger P, et al. Stromal expression of heat shock protein 27 is associated with worse clinical outcome in patients with colorectal cancer lung metastases. PLoS One 2015;20:e0120724.

45. Zink S, Kayser G, Gabius HJ, et al. Survival, disease free interval, and associated tumor features in patients with colon/rectal carcinomas and their resected intra-pulmonary metastases. Eur J Cardiothorac Surg 2001;19:908–13.

46. Rena O, Casadio C, Viano F, et al. Pulmonary resection for metastases from colorectal cancer: factors influencing prognosis. Twentyyear experience. Eur J Cardiothorac Surg 2002;21:906–12.

47. Saito Y, Omiya H, Kohno K, et al. Pulmonary metastasectomy for 165 patients with colorectal carcinoma: A prognostic assessment. J Thorac Cardiovasc Surg 2002;124:1007–13.

48. Pfannschmidt J, Muley T, Hoffmann H, et al. Prognostic factors and survival after complete resection of pulmonary metastases from colorectal carcinoma: experiences in 167 patients. J Thorac Cardiovasc Surg 2003;126:732–9.

49. Inoue M, Kotake Y, Nakagawa K, et al. Surgery for pulmonary metastases from colorectal carcinoma. Ann Thorac Surg 2000;70:380–3.

50. Melloni G, Doglioni C, Bandiera A, et al. Prognostic factors and analysis of microsatellite instability in resected pulmonary metastases from colorectal carcinoma. Ann Thorac Surg 2006;81:2008–13.

51. Yedibela S, Klein P, Feuchter K, et al. Surgical management of pulmonary metastases from colorectal cancer in 153 patients. Ann Surg Oncol 2006;13:1538–44.

52. Welter S, Jacobs J, Krbek T, et al. Prognostic impact of lymph node involvement in pulmonary metastases from colorectal cancer. Eur J Cardiothorac Surg 2007;31:67–172.

53. Lin BR, Chang TC, Lee YC, et al. Pulmonary resection for colorectal cancer metastases: duration between cancer onset and lung metastasis as an important prognostic factor. Ann Surg Oncol 2009;16:1026–32.

54. Onaitis MW, Petersen RP, Haney JC, et al. Prognostic factors for recurrence after pulmonary resection of colorectal cancer metastases. Ann Thorac Surg 2009;87:1684–8.

55. Watanabe K, Nagai K, Kobayashi A, et al. Factors influencing survival after complete resection of pulmonary metastases from colorectal cancer. Br J Surg 2009;96:1058–65.

56. Landes U, Robert J, Perneger T, et al. Predicting survival after pulmonary metastasectomy for colorectal cancer: previous liver metastases matter. BMC Surg 2010;10:17.

57. Riquet M, Foucault C, Cazes A, et al. Pulmonary resection for metastases of colorectal adenocarcinoma. Ann Thorac Surg 2010;89:375–80.

58. Zabaleta J, Aguinagalde B, Fuentes MG, et al. Survival after lung metastasectomy for colorectal cancer: importance of previous liver metastasis as a prognostic factor. Eur J Surg Oncol 2011;37:786–90.

Results of Pulmonary Resection
Sarcoma and Germ Cell Tumors

DuyKhanh P. Ceppa, MD

KEYWORDS

- Pulmonary metastasis • Lung resection • Sarcoma • Germ cell tumor • Outcomes

KEY POINTS

- Patients with controlled primary disease, absent extrathoracic disease, sufficient pulmonary function, and overall functional capacity with pulmonary metastases that can be completely resected are candidates for pulmonary metastatectomy.
- Patients undergoing pulmonary metastatectomy of osteosarcoma may have a 5-year survival of 35% to 50%; for patients undergoing resection of soft tissue sarcoma metastases it is 35% to 52%.
- Large case series of pulmonary metastatectomy of nonseminomatous germ cell tumor (NSGCT) have reported 5-year survival rates of greater than 80%.
- There are no randomized trials on pulmonary metastatectomy in patients with metastatic sarcoma or NSGCT; Survival rates are from case series.

INTRODUCTION: NATURE OF THE PROBLEM

Pulmonary metastatectomy dates back to the 1880s.[1] Sublobar resections, lobectomy, and pneumonectomy described were subsequently in the setting of metastatic sarcoma, renal cell cancer, and colon cancer.[2,3] Selection criteria for pulmonary metastatectomy were proposed formally in a case series of pulmonary metastatectomies by Alexander and Haight.[4] Since then, with increasing supportive data, pulmonary metastatectomy has become a widely accepted treatment modality for patients with metastatic disease.

As many as 88% of patients with sarcoma were found to have single-site pulmonary metastatic disease in a retrospective study by Huth and Eilber.[5] In a case series from Memorial Sloan-Kettering Cancer Center, Billingsley and colleagues[6] reported that 73% of 230 patients with recurrent soft tissue sarcoma had recurrences that initially appeared in the lungs. Eight percent of patients with clinical stage I nonseminomatous germ cell tumor (NSGCT) develop pulmonary metastases. Additionally, an estimated 10% to 20% of patients with stage III disease who were treated with cisplatin-based chemotherapy have residual intrathoracic disease requiring mediastinal dissection or pulmonary metastatectomy.[7] Pulmonary metastatectomy may be the only therapeutic option to render these patients disease free.

THERAPEUTIC OPTIONS AND SURGICAL TECHNIQUE

After systemic therapy and confirmation of limited disease, therapeutic options for controlled pulmonary metastases include continued systemic chemotherapy, isolated lung perfusion or suffusion, radiofrequency ablation, stereotactic body radiation therapy, and surgical resection. Isolated lung perfusion or suffusion, radiofrequency ablation, and stereotactic body radiation therapy are covered more thoroughly elsewhere in this issue.

The author has nothing to disclose.
Division of Cardiothoracic Surgery, Department of Surgery, Indiana University School of Medicine, 545 Barnhill Drive, EH215, Indianapolis, IN 46202, USA
E-mail address: dpceppa@iupui.edu

Thorac Surg Clin 26 (2016) 49–54
http://dx.doi.org/10.1016/j.thorsurg.2015.09.007
1547-4127/16/$ – see front matter © 2016 Elsevier Inc. All rights reserved.

Patients being considered for pulmonary metastatectomy should meet the following criteria: (1) controlled primary site of disease, (2) absence of extrathoracic metastases (or, in cases of oligometastases, extrathoracic sites of metastases are controlled or controllable), (3) sufficient pulmonary reserve to tolerate the proposed pulmonary resection, (4) completely resectable pulmonary metastatic disease with predictably sufficient pulmonary reserve. Preoperative planning should include pulmonary function testing and an evaluation of the patient's ability to tolerate an operation. Special consideration should be taken for patients receiving certain chemotherapeutic agents (bleomycin, mitomycin C, busulfan, cyclophosphamide, carmustine, gefitinib, paclitaxel, and methotrexate). These patients are at risk for drug-induced lung disease, including interstitial pneumonitis and fibrosis, hypersensitivity pneumonitis, and acute pneumonia. Fractional inspired oxygen should be minimized to minimize the risk of oxygen toxicity. Finally, patients should be required to engage in smoking cessation for at least 3 weeks before surgery to decrease the risk of postoperative pneumonia and other complications.

Pulmonary metastatectomy can be achieved via thoracoscopy or thoracotomy for unilateral disease. Patients with bilateral pulmonary metastases can undergo bilateral thoracoscopy/thoracotomy, median sternotomy, or bilateral transternal (clamshell) thoracotomy. Proponents of open resection argue that more pulmonary nodules can be identified with manual palpation.[8–11] The identification of more nodules, however, does not translate to improved survival,[12] and proponents of thoracoscopy argue that patients undergoing thoracotomy experience significantly more complications[11] but no greater ipsilateral resections. The European Society of Thoracic Surgeons working group addressed several key issues to take into consideration in this decision-making process.[12] The European Society of Thoracic Surgeons considers open and thoracoscopic approaches equivalent, advising that surgeons should use their most trusted technique. Additionally, there are no data demonstrating a difference in outcome between an initial policy of bilateral versus unilateral exploration or simultaneous versus a staged approach in patients with known bilateral disease. Results from the European Society of Thoracic Surgeons working group survey suggested that an initial approach via median sternotomy is acceptable. In cases not suitable for median sternotomy—such as posterior lesions or patients with previous pulmonary resection—staged thoracotomy with a 3- to 6-week interval was recommended. Zheng and Fernando[13]

recommended a similar approach to pulmonary metastatectomy, except that these authors were more supportive of a thoracoscopic approach.

Ultimately, the main principle of surgical resection of pulmonary metastases is complete resection. When possible, preservation of pulmonary function should be maximized by limiting resection. Peripheral nodules can be treated with a wedge resection. More central nodules may require a segmentectomy or lobectomy. Very rarely, a pneumonectomy may be necessary and appropriate to achieve complete resection.

CLINICAL OUTCOMES
Sarcoma

In a study by the Cooperative Osteosarcoma Study group, 81% of patients with sarcoma presenting with metastatic disease had pulmonary metastases.[14] Sixty-two percent of these patients have metastatic disease in the lungs only. Because sarcoma often does not respond to systemic or radiation therapy, complete resection with a pulmonary metastatectomy may be the only means by which to render a patient with single-site sarcoma metastasis free of disease.

There are few prospective studies and no randomized trials evaluating the role of pulmonary metastatectomy in the management of patients with osteogenic sarcoma. The first significant case series was described by Martini and associates,[15] who describe 22 patients who collectively underwent 59 procedures for the resection of 152 nodules. The authors reported a 3-year survival rate of 45%. Similarly, in subsequent case series, Snyder and colleagues[16] and Putnam and colleagues[17] in their series of 21 and 39 patients, respectively, both reported 5-year survival rates of nearly 40% in patients with osteogenic sarcoma who underwent pulmonary metastatectomy. The presence of 3 or fewer nodules on preoperative imaging was found to be the single most useful preoperative risk factor.

In more recent case series, Kim and colleagues[18] published their results in 97 patients who underwent pulmonary metastatectomy between June 2002 and December 2008. They reported an overall 5-year survival of 50.1% and noted that patients with a disease-free interval less than 12 months ($P = .001$), 2 or more pulmonary metastases ($P = .0007$), a lesion greater than 3 cm in diameter ($P = .017$), and a positive resection margin ($P = .004$) had significantly worse survival. Conversely, histology, tumor grade, and use of chemotherapy were found to have no effect on survival. Another series analyzed the outcomes of 47 patients with osteosarcoma. This study found that on multivariable analysis age greater than 45 years, a disease-free interval of greater than 1 year, synchronous disease, thoracotomy, histology, and performance of lobectomy were associated with poor overall survival.[19] Moreover, patients with an increasing number of risk factors were associated with a poor overall survival (64% at 5 years for patients with 3 risk factors vs 3% at 5 years for patients with 5 risk factors). Finally, a multiinstitutional review of 39 pediatric cases of metastatic osteosarcoma presenting with pulmonary metastases more than 1 year after primary site diagnosis reported a postresection event free survival of 33% at 5 years and postresection survival of 56.8% at 5 years.[20] These authors concluded that long-term survivors in patients who presented with pulmonary metastases are possible (53% postresection overall survival at 10 years). They endorsed pulmonary metastatectomy and reported that the addition chemotherapy did not add benefit.

Patients with soft tissue sarcoma are distinct from those with osteosarcoma. Approximately 23% of patients with soft tissue sarcoma develop distant metastases.[6] As with osteosarcoma, the lung is the most common metastatic site, accounting for up to 80% of metastases.[21] Pulmonary metastatectomy, similarly, represents the only potentially curative treatment for patients with soft tissue sarcoma and pulmonary dissemination.[22,23]

The first soft tissue sarcoma pulmonary metastatectomy was described by Weinlechner, at which time 2 incidentally found lesions were removed during a resection of a chest wall sarcoma.[24] Since then, Van Geel and Sardenberg and their colleagues have published their case series. van Geel and colleagues[25] reported a 5-year survival of 38% for patients with soft tissue sarcoma undergoing pulmonary metastatectomy in their case series of 255 patients. Sardenberg and associates[26] reported a 7.5-year survival rate of 34.7%. Finally, Predina and colleagues[27] reported 3- and 5-year overall survival rates of 67% and 52%, respectively, from their series of 48 patients undergoing metastatectomy for soft tissue sarcoma. The authors do concede that their improved results compared with historical controls were likely owing to careful patient selection. As with other primary sites, a longer disease-free interval (>6 months) and fewer than 3 nodules are associated with a higher overall 5-year survival. Repeated pulmonary metastatectomy was also associated with improved survival.[28,29] However, patients with soft tissue sarcoma presenting with synchronous pulmonary metastasis were not found to benefit from metastatectomy, and thus should be considered for clinical trials.[30,31]

Treasure and colleagues[32] performed a systematic review of published case series on pulmonary metastatectomy for sarcoma. Eighteen studies published between 1991 and 2010 were included, involving 1357 patients, 43% of whom underwent subsequent metastatectomy. The reported 5-year survival for patients with osteosarcoma was 34%. The reported 5-year survival for patients with soft tissue sarcoma was 25%. In comparison, the 5-year survival reported from data from the Thames Cancer Registry was 20% to 25% and 13% to 15% in patients with bone sarcoma and soft tissue sarcoma, respectively. Improved survival was associated with the presence of fewer metastatic lesion and longer disease-free intervals. The authors, however, were very explicit in stating that there was no evidence to support that survival improvement was attributable to metastatectomy because there were no controls nor was treatment randomized in any of the studies included in the review. They proposed that improved patient survival was a result of patient selection and not an effect of metastatectomy. Aberg and coworkers published similar views previously.[33,34] The authors emphasize the need for randomized trials to determine the true, and not the perceived, effect of pulmonary metastatectomy.

Germ Cell Tumors

When discussing pulmonary metastatectomy for germ cell tumors, it is typically in reference to NSGCT. Metastatectomy in seminoma has a limited role, but has been advocated in the setting of residual masses 3 cm or larger.[35] This is on account of the fact that viable disease or relapse in patients with seminoma has been noted in cases with residual masses 3 cm or larger at a rate of 27%, compared with a rate of 3% in cases with residual masses less than 3 cm or no residual masses on computed tomography.[36] There are no reliable survival data on pulmonary metastatectomy for seminoma, however. The practice at Indiana University is to follow patients with residual disease with serial computed tomography, considering surgical intervention only for patients with growth of the residual mass in patients with teratoma on testicular pathology. Conversely, pulmonary metastatectomy in NSGCT is widely accepted with good long-term results. In fact, data from the International Registry of Lung Metastasis identified patients with germ cell tumors ($P = .04$) as being associated with a better prognosis than patients with pulmonary metastases from other malignancies.

Owing to excellent results from effective chemotherapy regimens, pulmonary metastatectomy for

NSGCT currently serves an adjunct role in the treatment of patients with metastatic NSGCT. All patients with persistent pulmonary nodules on radiologic imaging after systemic therapy should be considered for resection. However, only 5% to 10% of patients with metastatic NSGCT require pulmonary metastatectomy.[37] Steyerberg and colleagues[38] reported that histology at residual retroperitoneal lymph node dissection (RPLND) was a strong predictor of histology at thoracotomy. However, several authors have reported pathology from residual RPLND to differ from pathology from residual pulmonary nodules in as high as 30% of cases.[39–42] Therefore, pulmonary metastatectomy should be considered even in cases with necrosis or fibrosis on RPLND.

Five-year survival rates of up to 79% to 87% were reported in early, small case series.[39,41,42] Liu and colleauges[43] from Memorial Sloan-Kettering Cancer Center published the first single-institution large case series of 157 patients undergoing pulmonary metastatectomy for germ cell tumor (between July 1967 and May 1995). Forty-four percent of patients had viable tumor in the resected specimen, and 26% of patients had metastases to other sites. Overall 5-year survival after pulmonary resection was 68%, but 82% for patients diagnosed after 1985, when cisplatin-based chemotherapy regimens for NSGCT were introduced.[43] Persistent carcinoma in the specimen ($P<.0001$), and concurrent metastases to nonpulmonary, visceral sites ($P = .0069$) were negative prognostic factors.

In 2005, Kesler and colleagues[44] reported Indiana University's series of patients with metastatic NSGCT, 59 and 26 of whom had pulmonary metastases and both mediastinal and pulmonary metastases, respectively, as salvage therapy. Median survival was 5.6 years, and it was reported that after a mean follow-up of 5.1 years, 42.3% of patients were alive and without disease. Older age, pulmonary metastases (vs mediastinal metastases), and 4 or more total intrathoracic lesions were found to be significantly predictive of worse long-term survival. In 2011, Kesler, and colleagues[45] reported the complete series of 159 patients undergoing pulmonary metastatectomy and 136 patients undergoing both pulmonary and mediastinal metastatectomy. More than one-half of patients (52.7%) were noted to have teratoma, 21.5% had necrosis, 15% persistent NSGCT, and 10.1% degenerative non–germ cell cancer. Median survival was 23.5 years and more than 68% of patients were alive without disease after a mean of 5.6 years. Older age at diagnosis ($P = .001$), non–germ cell cancer in testes specimen ($P = .004$), and residual disease ($P<.001$)

were significantly predictive of survival. Survival was the same in patients with hematogenous versus lymphatic metastases. Finally, the authors reported that residual pathology was the driving predictor of survival.

Simultaneous pulmonary metastatectomy and RPLND can be performed with acceptable morbidity and mortality in selected patients.[46] Similarly, pulmonary metastatectomy via staged thoracotomy or clamshell thoracotomy has been described for bilateral pulmonary disease with low morbidity. However, Besse and colleagues[47] suggests that, under certain circumstances, bilateral exploration could be avoided. The authors reported their results from a multiinstitutional retrospective review of 71 patients with residual pulmonary lesion after cisplatin-based chemotherapy. Of 39 patients with bilateral pulmonary disease, 2 (5%) had discordant histologic results. Moreover, of 20 patients with necrosis on initial pulmonary metastatectomy, 1 (5%) had teratoma on the contralateral lung. The authors concluded that with 95% pathologic concordance rate between the 2 lungs, contralateral pulmonary metastatectomy could be avoided when complete necrosis is found on the initial side pulmonary resection.

COMPLICATIONS AND CONCERNS

Complete pulmonary metastatectomy can be achieved with low morbidity and mortality. Surgical mortality is akin to pulmonary resection for other diagnoses (0%–0.6%).[39,41–43] A surgical mortality of less than 1% was reported in pulmonary metastatectomy in the Indiana University series.[45] However, the majority of surgical mortalities were in patients undergoing simultaneous resection of pulmonary and mediastinal disease. The most commonly reported complications are pneumonia, respiratory failure, atrial fibrillation, prolonged air leak, and prolonged ventilation.[19] Chyle leaks can also occur in patients with NSGCT who are concurrently undergoing an extensive lymphadenectomy for residual mediastinal NSGCT lesions.[45]

SUMMARY

Pulmonary metastatectomy plays a central role in the treatment of patients with metastatic sarcoma and germ cell tumors. Five-year survival rates can be as high as 50% for patients with sarcoma and 80% for patients with NSGCT. These survival rates are significantly improved compared with historical controls. Current data in support of pulmonary metastatectomy for sarcoma and NSGCT, however, are derived from nonrandomized case series without observation controls. Therefore, the reported survival rates could be a reflection of patient selection bias as opposed to the true curative effect of pulmonary metastatectomy. Randomized trials (in a multiinstitutional effort) need to be performed.

REFERENCES

1. Dominguez-Ventura A, Nichols FC 3rd. Lymphade-nectomy in metastasectomy. Thorac Surg Clin 2006;16(2):139–43.
2. Barney JD, Churchill E. Adenocarcinoma of the kidney with metastasis to the lung cured by ne-phrectomy and lobectomy. J Urol 1939;42:269.
3. Pastorino U, Treasure T. A historical note on pulmo-nary metastasectomy. J Thorac Oncol 2010; 5(6 Suppl 2):S132–3.
4. Alexander J, Haight C. Pulmonary resection for solitary metastatic sarcomas and carcinomas. Surg Gynecol Obstet 1947;85(2):129–46.
5. Huth JF, Eilber FR. Patterns of recurrence after resection of osteosarcoma of the extremity. Strate-gies for treatment of metastases. Arch Surg 1989; 124(1):122–6.
6. Billingsley KG, Lewis JJ, Leung DH, et al. Multifacto-rial analysis of the survival of patients with distant metastasis arising from primary extremity sarcoma. Cancer 1999;85(2):389–95.
7. Kesler KA, Donohue JP. Combined urologic and thoracic approaches for advanced or disseminated testis cancer. Atlas of Urol Clin N Am 1999;7:79–94.
8. McCormack PM, Bains MS, Begg CB, et al. Role of video-assisted thoracic surgery in the treatment of pul-monary metastases: results of a prospective trial. Ann Thorac Surg 1996;62(1):213–6 [discussion: 216–7].
9. Cerfolio RJ, McCarty T, Bryant AS. Non-imaged pulmonary nodules discovered during thoracotomy for metastasectomy by lung palpation. Eur J Cardio-thorac Surg 2009;35(5):786–91 [discussion: 791].
10. Kayton ML, Huvos AG, Casher J, et al. Computed tomographic scan of the chest underestimates the number of metastatic lesions in osteosarcoma. J Pediatr Surg 2006;41(1):200–6 [discussion: 200–6].
11. Mutsaerts EL, Zoetmulder FA, Meijer S, et al. Long term survival of thoracoscopic metastasectomy vs metastasectomy by thoracotomy in patients with a solitary pulmonary lesion. Eur J Surg Oncol 2002; 28(8):864–8.
12. Molnar TF, Gebitekin C, Turna A. What are the con-siderations in the surgical approach in pulmonary metastasectomy? J Thorac Oncol 2010;5(6 Suppl 2):S140–4.
13. Zheng Y, Fernando HC. Surgical and nonresectional therapies for pulmonary metastasis. Surg Clin North Am 2010;90(5):1041–51.
14. Kager L, Zoubek A, Potschger U, et al. Primary met-astatic osteosarcoma: presentation and outcome of patients treated on neoadjuvant Cooperative Osteo-sarcoma Study Group protocols. J Clin Oncol 2003; 21(10):2011–8.
15. Martini N, Huvos AG, Mike V, et al. Multiple pulmo-nary resections in the treatment of osteogenic sar-coma. Ann Thorac Surg 1971;12(3):271–80.
16. Snyder CL, Saltzman DA, Ferrell KL, et al. A new approach to the resection of pulmonary osteo-sarcoma metastases. Results of aggressive metasta-sectomy. Clin Orthop Relat Res 1991;(270):247–53.
17. Putnam JB Jr, Roth JA, Wesley MN, et al. Survival following aggressive resection of pulmonary metas-tases from osteogenic sarcoma: analysis of prognostic factors. Ann Thorac Surg 1983;36(5): 516–23.
18. Kim S, Ott HC, Wright CD, et al. Pulmonary resection of metastatic sarcoma: prognostic factors associ-ated with improved outcomes. Ann Thorac Surg 2011;92(5):1780–6 [discussion: 1786–7].
19. Lin AY, Kotova S, Yanagawa J, et al. Risk stratifica-tion of patients undergoing pulmonary metastasec-tomy for soft tissue and bone sarcomas. J Thorac Cardiovasc Surg 2015;149(1):85–92.
20. Daw NC, Chou AJ, Jaffe N, et al. Recurrent osteosar-coma with a single pulmonary metastasis: a multi-institutional review. Br J Cancer 2015;112(2):278–82.
21. Potter DA, Glenn J, Kinsella T, et al. Patterns of recurrence in patients with high-grade soft-tissue sarcomas. J Clin Oncol 1985;3(3):353–66.
22. Temple LK, Brennan MF. The role of pulmonary metastasectomy in soft tissue sarcoma. Semin Thorac Cardiovasc Surg 2002;14(1):35–44.
23. King JJ, Fayssoux RS, Lackman RD, et al. Early out-comes of soft tissue sarcomas presenting with me-tastases and treated with chemotherapy. Am J Clin Oncol 2009;32(3):308–13.
24. Smith RD. Pulmonary metastatectomy for soft tissue sarcoma. Surg Oncol Clin N Am 2012;21:269–86.
25. van Geel AN, Pastorino U, Jauch KW, et al. Surgical treatment of lung metastases: the European Organi-zation for Research and Treatment of Cancer-Soft Tissue and Bone Sarcoma Group study of 255 pa-tients. Cancer 1996;77(4):675–82.
26. Sardenberg RA, Figueiredo LP, Haddad FJ, et al. Pulmonary metastasectomy from soft tissue sar-comas. Clinics (Sao Paulo) 2010;65(9):871–6.
27. Predina JD, Puc MM, Bergey MR, et al. Improved survival after pulmonary metastasectomy for soft tis-sue sarcoma. J Thorac Oncol 2011;6(5):913–9.
28. Burt BM, Ocejo S, Mery CM, et al. Repeated and aggressive pulmonary resections for leiomyosar-coma metastases extends survival. Ann Thorac Surg 2011;92(4):1202–7.
29. Pogrebniak HW, Roth JA, Steinberg SM, et al. Reo-perative pulmonary resection in patients with

metastatic soft tissue sarcoma. Ann Thorac Surg 1991;52(2):197–203.

30. Kane JM, Finley JW, Driscoll D, et al. The treatment and outcome of patients with soft tissue sarcomas and synchronous metastases. Sarcoma 2002;6(2): 69–73.

31. Ferguson PC, Deheshi BM, Chung P, et al. Soft tissue sarcoma presenting with metastatic disease: outcome with primary surgical resection. Cancer 2011;117(2):372–9.

32. Treasure T, Fiorentino F, Scarci M, et al. Pulmonary metastasectomy for sarcoma: a systematic review of reported outcomes in the context of Thames Cancer Registry data. BMJ Open 2012; 2(5). pii:e001736.

33. Aberg T. Selection mechanisms as major determinants of survival after pulmonary metastasectomy. Ann Thorac Surg 1997;63(3):611–2.

34. Aberg T, Malmberg KA, Nilsson B, et al. The effect of metastasectomy: fact or fiction? Ann Thorac Surg 1980;30(4):378–84.

35. Xiao H, Liu D, Bajorin DF, et al. Medical and surgical management of pulmonary metastases from germ cell tumors. Chest Surg Clin N Am 1998;8(1): 131–43.

36. Puc HS, Heelan R, Mazumdar M, et al. Management of residual mass in advanced seminoma: results and recommendations from the Memorial Sloan-Kettering Cancer Center. J Clin Oncol 1996;14(2): 454–60.

37. Boffa DJ, Rusch VW. Surgical techniques for nonseminomatous germ cell tumors metastatic to the lung. Chest Surg Clin N Am 2002;12(4):739–48.

38. Steyerberg EW, Donohue JP, Gerl A, et al. Residual masses after chemotherapy for metastatic testicular cancer: the clinical implications of the association between retroperitoneal and pulmonary histology. Re-analysis of Histology in Testicular Cancer (ReHiT) Study Group. J Urol 1997;158(2):474–8.

39. Gerl A, Clemm C, Schmeller N, et al. Sequential resection of residual abdominal and thoracic masses after chemotherapy for metastatic non-seminomatous germ cell tumours. Br J Cancer 1994;70(5):960–5.

40. Fizazi K, Tjulandin S, Salvioni R, et al. Viable malignant cells after primary chemotherapy for disseminated nonseminomatous germ cell tumors: prognostic factors and role of postsurgery chemotherapy–results from an international study group. J Clin Oncol 2001;19(10):2647–57.

41. Brenner PC, Herr HW, Morse MJ, et al. Simultaneous retroperitoneal, thoracic, and cervical resection of postchemotherapy residual masses in patients with metastatic nonseminomatous germ cell tumors of the testis. J Clin Oncol 1996;14(6):1765–9.

42. Gels ME, Hoekstra HJ, Sleijfer DT, et al. Thoracotomy for postchemotherapy resection of pulmonary residual tumor mass in patients with nonseminomatous testicular germ cell tumors: aggressive surgical resection is justified. Chest 1997;112(4):967–73.

43. Liu D, Abolhoda A, Burt ME, et al. Pulmonary metastasectomy for testicular germ cell tumors: a 28-year experience. Ann Thorac Surg 1998;66(5):1709–14.

44. Kesler KA, Wilson JL, Cosgrove JA, et al. Surgical salvage therapy for malignant intrathoracic metastases from nonseminomatous germ cell cancer of testicular origin: analysis of a single-institution experience. J Thorac Cardiovasc Surg 2005; 130(2):408–15.

45. Kesler KA, Kruter LE, Perkins SM, et al. Survival after resection for metastatic testicular nonseminomatous germ cell cancer to the lung or mediastinum. Ann Thorac Surg 2011;91(4):1085–93 [discussion: 1093].

46. Mandelbaum I, Yaw PB, Einhorn LH, et al. The importance of one-stage median sternotomy and retroperitoneal node dissection in disseminated testicular cancer. Ann Thorac Surg 1983;36(5): 524–8.

47. Besse B, Grunenwald D, Flechon A, et al. Nonseminomatous germ cell tumors: assessing the need for postchemotherapy contralateral pulmonary resection in patients with ipsilateral complete necrosis. J Thorac Cardiovasc Surg 2009;137(2):448–52.

Isolated Lung Perfusion for Pulmonary Metastases

Alison Ward, MD, Kirill Prokrym, BA, Harvey Pass, MD*

KEYWORDS

- Isolated lung perfusion • Pulmonary metastasis • Pulmonary artery perfusion • Chemotherapy

KEY POINTS

- Isolated lung perfusion (ILP) for pulmonary metastasis allows the lung to be preferentially perfused with high doses of chemotherapy, avoiding the dose-limiting effects of systemic toxicity.
- ILP can be performed retrograde or antegrade, with hyperthermia, using a blood flow occlusion technique, or using delayed clamp release. Minimally invasive techniques may be used.
- Doxorubicin, 5-flurodeoxyuridine, tumor necrosis factor alpha, paclitaxel, melphalan, gemcitabine, and cisplatin have all been used in ILP for pulmonary metastases.
- Several small and large animal models have been developed showing safety and reproducibility of ILP.
- Several phase I clinical trials showed ILP to be feasible in patients with pulmonary metastases, but long-term outcomes and survival are mixed.

INTRODUCTION

The lung is the most common site of metastatic involvement for invasive cancer, largely because circulating tumor cells are filtered via the pulmonary capillary bed. The incidence of lung metastases varies with tumor type and time of diagnosis of the primary cancer. Some cancers, such as sarcomas, often metastasize to the lungs with 20% to 30% of patients with metastatic cancer experiencing secondary spread to the lung.[1] Lung metastases are treated commonly using surgical resection, a technique with 5-year survival rates of only 20% to 40%.[2] Many patients experience recurrent pulmonary disease from micrometastases unrecognized at the time of pulmonary resection. Although reoperation for recurrent pulmonary metastases is an option, many patients are poor surgical candidates owing to lack of adequate pulmonary reserve or poor functional status. When lung metastases are inoperable, most patients die within 1 year.[2] Intravenous (IV) chemotherapy, another common treatment option for cancer, is limited by systemic side effects and toxicity, failing to significantly prolong patient survival.[2] Poor results seem to be attributed to drug resistance within the tumor mass and inability to deliver effective drug concentrations owing to systemic side effects and toxicity associated with higher doses.[1]

Isolated lung perfusion (ILP) is a surgical technique developed to deliver high-dose chemotherapy to the lung, minimizing systemic exposure by selectively delivering agent though the pulmonary artery and selectively diverting venous effluent. ILP has the distinct advantage of delivering high-dose drug treatment to the lung while limiting exposure of sensitive critical organs, thus avoiding severe complications. In addition, ILP minimizes the impact of active drug loss from renal metabolism of the drugs.[1] The lung was identified as an ideal organ for isolated perfusion because of its symmetry, an exclusive arterial supply from the pulmonary artery, venous drainage into 2 pulmonary veins (PV), and tolerance for hyperthermic conditions without significantly impairing systemic function.[3–5]

First proposed in 1958 by Creech and colleagues[6] testing nitrogen mustard in different

Department of Cardiothoracic Surgery, NYU Langone Medical Center, 530 First Avenue, New York, NY 10016, USA
* Corresponding author.
E-mail address: harvey.pass@nyumc.org

Thorac Surg Clin 26 (2016) 55–67
http://dx.doi.org/10.1016/j.thorsurg.2015.09.008

organs, ILP was developed originally to convert inoperable pulmonary metastases into resectable malignancies. Current usage of ILP is aimed to treat micrometastatic disease and improve first-order targeting.[7] Most research regarding ILP has focused on sarcoma and colorectal carcinoma pulmonary metastases. Notably, Johnston and associates[8] began research into ILP in 1983, investigating the toxicity and pharmacokinetics of doxorubicin in addition to the effect of hyperthermia on lung function and uptake of doxorubicin during ILP. Johnston and colleagues[8] described a staged bilateral isolated single lung and simultaneous bilateral lung perfusion in dogs and humans, providing initial data on the technique's safety and reproducibility. Other groups have described results using various chemotherapeutic drugs, including: doxorubicin, liposomal-encapsulated doxorubicin (Liporubicin), 5-flurodeoxyuridine (FUDR), tumor necrosis factor alpha (TNF-α), paclitaxel, melphalan, gemcitabine, combined use of gemcitabine and carboplatin, and cisplatin. Studies examined in this retrospective article include assay, cellular, rat, dog, pig, sheep, and human phase I models in evaluation of ILP as a feasible and reproducible surgical technique.

SURGICAL TECHNIQUE

The premise behind ILP for pulmonary metastasis is that the lung can be perfused preferentially with high doses of chemotherapy to the tumor while avoiding systemic toxicity. The lung is an ideal organ for this technique because it receives its arterial blood supply almost exclusively from the pulmonary artery (PA) and drains into the 2 PV.[5]

This nearly eliminates systemic toxicity while providing targeted therapy for both macroscopic disease and microscopic disease.

The patient is anesthetized, a double-lumen endotracheal tube is placed, and the patient is placed in a lateral position. A Swan–Ganz catheter is placed by some surgeons in the PA contralateral to the lung being perfused. An anterolateral or posterolateral thoracotomy is made and, if a Swan–Ganz catheter was placed, the position of the catheter is confirmed with palpation and adjusted as necessary. The pleural cavity is inspected to rule out extrapulmonary disease. Next, a pericardiotomy is made and the posterior mediastinum is dissected, ligating or occluding all systemic–pulmonary collaterals.[9–13] Some surgeons place an occluder around the main bronchus for occlusion of bronchial arteries.[12,13] The main PA and superior and inferior PV are dissected free. The patient is then systemically heparinized before occlusion of the PA and PV with vascular clamps. Two polypropylene purse-string sutures are placed in the PA and PV. Next, the cannulas are inserted. The arterial cannulas are placed in the main PA or a branch of the PA and the venous cannulas are placed in the superior and/or inferior PV and connected to the extracorporeal circuit to drain into the venous reservoir.[9–13]

The extracorporeal circuit, which is similar to the heart–lung machine used in cardiac surgical procedures, consists of a centrifugal or roller pump, membrane oxygenator, and heat exchanger. The perfusion circuit is primed before starting ILP.

There are 2 basic perfusion techniques—a single pass (Fig. 1) and a recirculating blood circuit. The single pass removes the venous effluent after

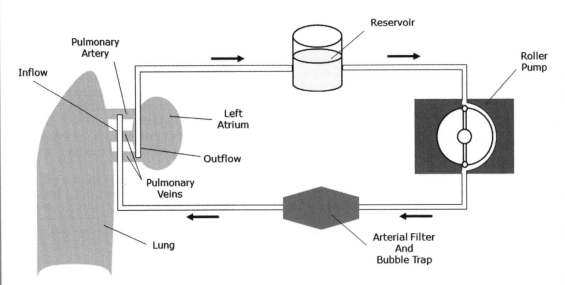

Fig. 1. Diagram of the perfusion circuit.

circulating the chemotherapeutic agent through the lung 1 time versus a recirculating blood circuit that collects the effluent and redelivers the drug to the lung.[5]

After ILP is complete, the lung is flushed with normothermic saline, Voluven, lactated Ringer's solution, or Hespan. After complete washout, the PA and PV cannulas are removed, protamine sulfate is given, hemostasis is achieved, and the vessels closed.[9–13]

Variations of the Isolated Lung Perfusion Technique

Antegrade versus retrograde perfusion
In the majority of published studies on ILP, chemotherapy is perfused into the lung in an antegrade technique via the PA. An alternative means of perfusion is in a retrograde manner via the superior and inferior PV. The effluent is then drained from the PV for antegrade and from the PA for retrograde perfusion. The proposed benefit behind retrograde perfusion is that, by perfusing through the PV, collaterals between the pulmonary and bronchial venous systems can be exploited to deliver drugs to the metastatic lesions.[14,15]

Blood flow occlusion technique
Furrer and colleagues[16] first described the blood flow occlusion (BFO) technique in a pig model. The procedure starts using the same technique as described, except that there is no need to dissect and isolate the PV. The PA is isolated, clamped, and a perfusion catheter is placed. The lung is perfused with continuous PA perfusion and the lung is ventilated simultaneously. Van Putte and colleagues[17] later described a similar model in rats.

Endovascular Blood Flow Occlusion Technique

This technique was described in a pig model as a possible alternative to the previously discussed methods of ILP that require a thoracotomy. The authors noted that this endovascular technique may be especially advantageous for patients needing repeated surgeries. A balloon tip catheter is introduced percutaneously into the right femoral vein. The catheter is advanced into the proximal left PA under fluoroscopic guidance and the PA is subsequently occluded upon inflation of the balloon. Angiography is performed to confirm correct positioning. Next, perfusion is initiated. After perfusion is complete, a repeat angiogram is performed to confirm the correct position of the PA catheter.[12,14]

Delayed Clamp Release

Delayed clamp release was developed to assess whether postponing flushing after ILP could limit drug washout and thereby maintain drug levels in the lung. Van Putte and colleagues evaluated the effect of using delayed clamp release in rats on gemcitabine lung levels after perfusion. ILP with gemcitabine was performed, followed by delayed clamp release of varying lengths of time and this was compared with the lung gemcitabine levels to those in rats who underwent ILP with the same amount of gemcitabine but with varying lengths of washout. The delayed clamp release resulted in significantly higher lung levels compared with traditional ILP with immediate washout.[15]

Selective Pulmonary Artery Perfusion

Selective PA perfusion (SPAP) is another endovascular technique used to deliver selective perfusion. First, a balloon-tipped catheter is introduced percutaneously into the left internal jugular vein. The balloon is positioned in the left PA under pressure guidance. A left anterolateral thoracotomy is made and the left PA is dissected free. The position of the balloon is confirmed with palpation. The tip of the catheter is positioned in the left main PA. Next, a flow probe is placed around the left PA for blood flow measurements. The balloon is inflated to achieve varying levels of flow reduction. In a study by Van Putte and colleagues, gemcitabine was then infused through the catheter. This method resulted in higher levels of gemcitabine within the lung without causing elevated levels in liver or serum when compared with IV administration. They did note that with blood flow reduction, drug distribution in the lung was not homogeneous.[16] In a subsequent study, the authors found that SPAP followed by BFO resulted in higher levels of gemcitabine in lung tissue and less variable distribution than SPAP with concomitant BFO.[17]

Hyperthermia

Many chemotherapeutic agents, including doxorubicin, bleomycin, mitomycin C, and cisplatin, have enhanced cytotoxic effects at higher temperatures.[9] Patient response has been promising in several papers comparing the use of hyperthermic versus normothermic perfusion.[9,15,18,19] The first clinical experience with hyperthermic ILP was described by Schröder and colleagues,[9] who developed a surgical technique for ILP with high doses of cisplatin under hyperthermic conditions (inflow temperature of $\geq 41^\circ C$) in 4 patients with recurrent or unresectable lung sarcoma metastases. In a pig model for hyperthermic ILP comparing low-dose normothermic cisplatin, hyperthermic perfusion, up to a temperature of $41.5^\circ C$, led to a reduction in the acute lung injury.[18]

In a follow-up in vivo large animal study, the influence of normothermic (38°C) and moderate hyperthermic (41.5°C) perfusion temperatures was addressed and hyperthermia was well-tolerated.[19] Another large animal model demonstrated that paclitaxel given by hyperthermic (39.5°C) retrograde ILP was feasible and well-tolerated. In in vitro studies, hyperthermia enhanced paclitaxel mediated toxicity in all cancer cells especially melanoma and sarcoma cell lines and no toxicity was seen in normal human bronchial epithelial cells.[15]

Video-Assisted Transcatheter Isolated Lung Perfusion

Video-assisted thoracoscopic surgery (VATS) has become a widely accepted, minimally invasive technique for treating various thoracic diseases with excellent outcomes. In 2005, Jinbo and colleagues[20] described a new technique of VATS ILP in canines. First, a 9F sheath was placed in the femoral vein and a 7.5F balloon occlusion catheter was positioned in the left PA under fluoroscopic guidance. Heparin was then administered and the balloon was inflated. A 10-mm port was introduced into the sixth intercostal space and a mini thoracotomy was created in the fourth intercostal space. Each PV was encircled with tape and an 8F drainage cannula was introduced into each of those PV under thoracoscopic guidance. The effluent was suctioned continuously out of these cannulas and not reperfused. ILP was performed for 20 minutes at a flow rate of 30 mL/min with cisplatin. After perfusion, the lungs were flushed for 5 minutes at the same flow rate. At the end of the procedure, the cannulas were removed and the chest was closed.

CLINICAL OUTCOMES
Doxorubicin

In 1989, Baciewicz and colleagues[21] studied the pharmacokinetics and lung toxicity of doxorubicin and the ideal dose for an in vivo ILP model in dogs (**Table 1**). One group served as a control with no doxorubicin in the perfusate and the remaining 5 groups had concentrations of doxorubicin ranging from 1.95 to 7.61 µg/mL in the perfusate. The final lung tissue concentrations increased with increasing dose of doxorubicin in the perfusate. Regression analysis showed a significant dose–response relationship for the final perfusate concentration and for the lung tissue level of doxorubicin. No doxorubicin was detectable in the systemic blood samples of any of the dogs. The authors concluded that using a dose level of up to 6 µg/mL in the perfusate can be performed with little lung injury, systemic toxicity, or adverse

clinical outcomes. In 1998, Furrer and colleagues[16] sought to compare modalities of lung perfusion with doxorubicin in a swine model—ILP, BFO, endovascular BFO, and IV. The lung tissue doxorubicin level at the end of BFO was 9 times higher than that achieved by IV infusion. Plasma levels were not detectable in the ILP group, 0 to 0.44 µg/mL in the BFO group and 0.31 to 0.84 µg/mL in the IV group. Levels did not differ between ILP and BFO techniques. In the endovascular BFO group, the procedure was performed successfully in all 3 animals and 1 month postoperatively lung tissue showed no cytostatic-induced changes.

In 2000, Burt and colleagues[10] conducted a phase I trial of ILP with doxorubicin for patients with unresectable sarcoma pulmonary metastases. Eight patients were enrolled, 7 patients were treated with 40 mg/m^2 or less, and 1 patient received 80 mg/m^2. There were no perioperative deaths; however, 6 patients died of disease on follow-up out to 28 months. Unfortunately, there were no partial or complete responses to treatment. Only 1 patient showed stabilization of the lesions in the perfused lung when compared with the contralateral lung. The authors concluded that ILP with doxorubicin might serve an adjuvant role to eradicate micrometastases before resection in patients with resectable disease.

Yan and colleagues[22] compared ILP with doxorubicin and ILP with liposomal-encapsulated doxorubicin in a rat model. Rats with a single sarcoma pulmonary metastasis underwent ILP with free and liposomal doxorubicin. Cheng and colleagues[23] further investigated liposomal doxorubicin ILP and compared it to IV infusion in a rat model. Rats with a single sarcoma pulmonary metastasis underwent ILP or IV administration of either 100 or 400 µg of free doxorubicin or liposomal doxorubicin.

5-Flurodeoxyuridine

Burt's group at Memorial Sloan Kettering Cancer Center in New York also performed 2 studies looking at ILP with FUDR. In the first study, 28 BDIX rats with colon adenocarcinoma induced lung metastases were divided into 5 groups. The initial study demonstrated that ILP with FUDR at a concentration of 14 mg/mL is effective in treating metastatic colon adenocarcinoma resulting in fewer tumor nodules as compared with IV FUDR.[24] In the second study, the same model of ILP was used, but studied the toxicity and pharmacokinetics of FUDR ILP. Animals perfused with FUDR doses of greater than 21 mg/mL of FUDR died perioperatively. All animals perfused with

Table 1
Summary of chemotherapeutic agents used in ILP studies

Title	Year	First Author	Chemo Agent	Model	In Vitro Studies	Target Tumor Type	Additional Techniques
Pharmacokinetics of Paclitaxel Administered by Hyperthermic Retrograde ILP Techniques	2002	Schrump	Paclitaxel	Sheep	Yes	None (sarcoma)	Hyperthermia
ILP With TNF for Pulmonary Metastases	1995	Pass	TNF-α	Human	—	Mixed	Interferon, moderate hyperthermia
ILP with Platinum in the Treatment of Pulmonary Metastases From Soft Tissue Sarcomas	1995	Ratto	Cisplatin	Human	—	Sarcoma	—
Relationship Between the Concentration of CDDP in Tumor and Tumor Size After ILP Treatment Experimental Study on Solitary Pulmonary Sarcoma Model in Rats	2000	Saeki	Cisplatin	Rat	—	Sarcoma	—
Increasing Drug Concentration in a Rat Lung Tumor Model by Combining ILP with Hypertensive Chemotherapy	2001	Matsuoka	Cisplatin	Rat	—	Sarcoma	—
Technique and Results of Hyperthermic ILP with High-Doses of Cisplatin for the Treatment of Surgically Relapsing or Unresectable Lung Sarcoma Mets	2002	Schröder	Cisplatin	Human	—	Sarcoma	Hyperthermia
Evaluation of ILP as Neoadjuvant Therapy of Lung Metastases Using a Novel in vivo pig model: II. High Dose Cisplatin is Well Tolerated by the Native Lung Tissue	2003	Franke	Cisplatin	Swine	—	None	Hyperthermia, high dose

(continued on next page)

Table 1
(continued)

Title	Year	First Author	Chemo Agent	Model	In Vitro Studies	Target Tumor Type	Additional Techniques
VATS Transcatheter Lung Perfusion Regional Chemotherapy	2005	Jinbo	Cisplatin	Canine	—	None	VATS
Endovascular Lung Perfusion Using High-Dose Cisplatin: Uptake and DNA Adduct Formation in an Animal Model	2004	Brown	Cisplatin	Swine	—	None	Endovascular, high dose
ILP with FUDR is an Effective Treatment for Colorectal Adenocarcinoma Lung Metastases in Rats	1994	Ng	FUDR	Rat	—	Colorectal adenocarcinoma	—
ILP with FUDR in the Rat: Pharmacokinetics and Survival	1996	Port	FUDR	Rat	—	Colorectal adenocarcinoma	—
ILP with Melphalan for the Treatment of Metastatic Pulmonary Sarcoma	1996	Nawata	Melphalan	Rat	—	Sarcoma	—
ILP for the Treatment of Pulmonary Metastases An Experimental Study in the Rat	1999	Van Schil	Melphalan	Rat	—	Adenocarcinoma	TNF, unilateral and bilateral
ILP with Melphalan for Resectable Lung Metastases: A Phase I Clinical Trial	2004	Hendricks	Melphalan	Human	—	Mixed	Surgical resection
ILP with Melphalan: Pharmacokinetics and Toxicity in a Pig Model	2006	Van Der Elst	Melphalan	Swine	—	None	—
Pharmacokinetics and Toxicity of ILP with Doxorubicin	1989	Baciewicz	Doxorubicin	Canine	—	None	—
Cytostatic Lung Perfusion by Use of an Endovascular Blood Flow Occlusion Technique	1998	Furrer	Doxorubicin	Swine	—	None	BFO, endoBFO
ILP for Patients with Unresectable Metastases From Sarcoma: A Phase I Trial	2000	Burt	Doxorubicin	Human	—	Sarcoma	—

Title	Year	Author	Drug	Animal		Tumor	Notes
A Validated Assay for Measuring Doxorubicin in Biologic Fluids and Tissues in an ILP Model: Matrix Effect and Heparin Interference Strongly Influence Doxorubicin Measurements	2003	Kümmerle	Doxorubicin	Swine, Rat	—	None	Pharmacokinetics
Distribution of Free and Liposomal Doxorubicin After ILP in a Sarcoma Model	2008	Yan	Doxorubicin	Rat	—	Sarcoma	Liposomal
Drug Uptake in a Rodent Sarcoma Model after IV Injection or ILP of Free/Liposomal Doxorubicin	2009	Cheng	Doxorubicin	Rat	—	Sarcoma	Liposomal
ILP with Gemcitabine in a Rat: Pharmacokinetics and Survival	2002	Van Putte	Gemcitabine	Rat	Yes	Adenocarcinoma	—
Pharmacokinetics After Pulmonary Artery Perfusion With Gemcitabine	2003	Van Putte	Gemcitabine	Rat	Yes	Adenocarcinoma	BFO
Modified Approach of Administering Cytostatics to the Lung: More Efficient ILP	2006	Van Putte	Gemcitabine	Rat	—	None	Delayed clamp release
Pharmacokinetics of Gemcitabine When Delivered by Selective Pulmonary Artery Perfusion for the Treatment of Lung Cancer	2008	Van Putte	Gemcitabine	Swine	—	None	SPAP
Selective Pulmonary Artery Perfusion for the Treatment of Primary Lung Cancer: Improved Drug Exposure of the Lung	2005	Van Putte	Gemcitabine	Swine	—	None	SPAP, carboplatin
Selective Pulmonary Artery Perfusion Followed by Blood Flow Occlusion: New Challenge for the Treatment of Pulmonary Malignancies	2009	Grootenboers	Gemcitabine	Swine	—	None	SPAP, BFO
ILP as an Adjuvant Treatment of Colorectal Cancer Lung Metastases: A Preclinical Study in a Pig Model	2013	Pagès	Gemcitabine	Swine	Yes	Colorectal adenocarcinoma	—
Acute and Delayed Toxicity of Gemcitabine Administered During ILP: a Pre-Clinical Dose-Escalation Study in Pigs	2014	Pagès	Gemcitabine	Swine	—	None	—

Abbreviations: BFO, blood flow occlusion; CDDP, cisplatin; endoBFO, endovascular blood flow occlusion; FUDR, 5-flurodeoxyuridine; ILP, isolated lung perfusion; Mets, metastases; SPAP, selective pulmonary artery perfusion; TNF, tumor necrosis factor; VATS, video-assisted thoracoscopic surgery.

21 mg/mL survived the operation and 73% (8/11) survived until the end of the experiment. A small amount of systemic leak was noted in all ILP, groups but it was not statistically different than IV serum levels. The study demonstrated that the maximum tolerated dose of FUDR delivered via ILP was 21 mg/mL and that this dose led to minimal lung toxicity and maximally elevated total lung FUDR and 5-fluoracil.[25]

Tumor Necrosis Factor Alpha

In 1995, Pass and colleagues[13] conducted a phase I trial looking at the safety and feasibility of ILP with TNF-α and interferon-γ. Patients with good performance status and unresectable pulmonary metastatic disease were eligible. Fifteen patients underwent 16 ILPs. The initial TNF-α dose used was 0.3 mg. Dose escalation was performed up to a level of 6 mg at moderate hyperthermia. Patients received 0.2 mg of recombinant interferon-γ on each of the 2 days before surgery. Flow rates were determined by a perfusion pressure that was kept at a physiologic level. The target tissue temperature for perfusion was between 38°C and 39.5°C. A leak rate of 10% was noted for one patient and almost all other perfusions had rates of 0%. One patient had a prolonged intubation and intensive care unit course that the authors attributed to his smoking history and preoperative chemotherapy, and not to TNF-α toxicity, because his peak serum levels were well below the limits of detection. Three partial responses were seen within 8 weeks of ILP; however, new nodules or regrowth appeared 7 to 9 months postoperatively. In all patients the non-perfused side exhibited stable or worsening disease by 8 weeks postoperatively.

Paclitaxel

Schrump and colleagues[15] describe a sheep model of retrograde ILP with escalating doses of paclitaxel and hyperthermia. Ten sheep underwent ILP, 1 of which received perfusate without paclitaxel. The perfusion was continued for 90 minutes after which the lung was flushed with 1 L of lactated Ringer solution. Paclitaxel concentrations in lung tissues increased nonlinearly with increasing doses and peaked between 60 to 90 minutes. Paclitaxel concentrations in the systemic circulation were undetectable at all perfusate doses and after restoration of circulation the levels remained undetectable or were extremely low. There was no severe immediate clinical toxicity; only mild transient bronchorrhea was seen in the high-dose ILP animals once the lung was reventilated. This study demonstrated that paclitaxel

can be administered via hyperthermic retrograde ILP without immediate toxicity and is able to deliver higher concentrations of drug to the pulmonary tissues as compared with IV administration. In an in vitro study, hyperthermia enhanced paclitaxel-mediated toxicity in all cancer cells, especially melanoma and sarcoma cell lines, and no toxicity was seen in normal human bronchial epithelial cells.

Melphalan

In 1996, Nawata and colleagues[26] described a rat model with pulmonary metastatic sarcoma. ILP proceeded for 20 minutes with melphalan followed by a 10-minute washout at a rate of 0.5 mg/min. In this study, all rats perfused with greater than 2 mg of melphalan died. Rats perfused with 2 mg of melphalan survived pneumonectomy 67% of the time and those undergoing control ILP survived pneumonectomy 80% of the time. Animals that received ILP had significantly fewer left lung lesions as compared with animals given IV melphalan. In another rat model, Van Schil and colleagues[27] studied ILP with melphalan and TNF in comparison with IV melphalan for treatment of pulmonary metastatic adenocarcinoma. They found that, after ILP of the left lung, melphalan levels were significantly higher in that lung as compared with levels in the IV group and there were significantly fewer left lung nodules. TNF did not show any significant effect. They also showed that rats undergoing ILP with melphalan had significantly longer median survival and remained disease free.

In 2004, Hendriks and colleagues[12] conducted a phase I trial for ILP with melphalan. There were a total of 16 patients divided into 8 groups, all of whom had pulmonary metastases from melphalan-sensitive tumors. There were no operative or postoperative mortalities. Two patients who received 60 mg melphalan at 37°C developed lung edema and radiographic findings resembling a chemical pneumonitis. During the long-term follow-up, 7 of 16 patients had recurrent disease; 4 of 7 had disease outside of the lung and 1 of 7 were in the previously perfused lung. Van der Elst and colleagues[28] analyzed the pharmacokinetics and toxicity of melphalan ILP in a swine model. After the start of ILP, perfusate levels of melphalan remained stable and then declined rapidly after washout.

Gemcitabine

Van Putte and colleagues[29] have performed multiple studies with ILP using gemcitabine for treatment of colorectal adenocarcinoma pulmonary metastases. In 2002, they performed an in vitro and in vivo study. ILP of the left lung was performed for 25 minutes followed by 5 minutes of washout with buffered starch at a rate of 0.5 mL/min. ILP with either 160 or 320 mg/kg resulted in significantly higher left lung gemcitabine levels compared with those rats treated with IV 160 mg/kg. No gemcitabine was detected in the systemic circulation after ILP. The authors note that all animals died after IV infusion of 320 mg/kg. However, all animals survived with doses of up to 320 mg/kg via ILP demonstrating that ILP is less toxic than IV infusion. Next they evaluated BFO as a regional therapy with gemcitabine, again in a rat model. Compared with ILP, a higher nontoxic systemic exposure was present after BFO, whereas no different lung levels were seen for a lower total amount of gemcitabine given.[17] A follow-up study examined gemcitabine uptake in the lung at different inflow concentrations and the effect of delayed clamp release after ILP on lung levels. The authors concluded that ILP for 6 minutes with 6.7 mg/mL gemcitabine, followed by delayed clamp release for 30 minutes achieved as effective lung levels of gemcitabine compared with a standard 30-minute ILP.[30]

Van Putte and colleagues[31] also developed a swine catheterization model of SPAP combining the properties of ILP with IV treatment to achieve higher local drug levels and equivalent systemic exposure. SPAP for 2 and 10 minutes resulted in significantly higher lung levels when compared with IV, with 10 minutes achieving the highest level. The authors recommend using SPAP to downgrade primary lung tumors before surgical treatment. A series of studies investigated BFO after SPAP and dose escalation to delay washout of gemcitabine from lung tissue as well as a comparison of gemcitabine and carboplatin via SPAP (followed by BFO) or central venous line (IV).[32,33]

Pagès and associates[34] performed a series of investigations with ILP in a swine model with increasing doses of gemcitabine concentration of 0 to 640 µg/mL. Overall, 11 of 23 pigs were alive at 1 month. Immediate toxicity on lung parenchyma was seen with doses of 640 µg/mL and greater, including interstitial and alveolar infiltration with the extent of damage increasing with increasing doses. For this reason, the authors defined dose-limiting toxicity at 640 µg/mL and the maximum tolerated dose was set at 320 µg/mL.[35]

Cisplatin

In 1996, Ratto and colleagues[11] performed ILP in 6 patients with lung metastases from sarcoma. A dose of 200 mg/m² of cisplatin was used based on the highest dose used in an experimental model from previous studies. The authors were able to complete all procedures with no complications intraoperatively; there were no intraoperative or postoperative deaths. In 2 of 6 cases, a "contusion syndrome" occurred—radiographic signs of interstitial and alveolar edema. One of these patients needed 5 days of respiratory support. At 13 months, 4 of 6 patients were alive without evidence of disease recurrence. One patient died of extrapulmonary metastases and 1 patient had distant disease relapse. Chemotherapy toxicity occurred in none of the patients. The authors note that, instead of systemic toxicity limiting ILP, lung toxicity is likely the limiting factor. Additionally, they performed staged lung perfusion on 2 patients with bilateral disease and determined it was safe.[11]

In a second human study performed by Schröder and colleagues,[9] 4 patients with sarcoma lung metastases underwent ILP with high-dose cisplatin and hyperthermia. Two of these patients had bilateral disease. The operation was performed through posterolateral thoracotomy. Pulmonary metastectomy using a wedge resection or segmentectomy was performed before ILP to avoid misidentification of lesions from ILP induced fluid overload. Three patients were alive and disease free at 12 months. The fourth patient died from cerebral metastases without evidence of local disease recurrence.

In a swine model, Franke and colleagues[19] performed ILP with high-dose cisplatin under hyperthermic conditions. ILP was maintained for 40 minutes at normothermia followed by 5 minutes of washout. The perfusion was gradually increased up to a rate of 800 to 1000 mL/min and the lung was ventilated. They concluded that a cisplatin perfusate concentration of about 80 µg/mL (dose of about 300 mg/m²) is the dose limit of normothermic ILP. Hyperthermia tended to cause less acute lung injury, but this did not reach statistical significance. Saeki and colleagues[36] examined the pharmacokinetics of ILP using cisplatin in a rat solitary tumor model. The rats were divided into 12 groups, each subjected to varying durations of ILP and cisplatin concentrations. All of the animals tolerated ILP up to the maximum duration tested of 60 minutes. Higher concentrations were seen in smaller nodules, suggesting that ILP could be more effective against small tumors.

In 2004, Brown and colleagues[37] described a model for endovascular lung perfusion (ELP) with cisplatin in a swine model. Twelve swine were used; 6 underwent ELP with 150 mg cisplatin into the PA via a balloon occlusion catheter and 6 received 50 mg cisplatin IV. At all time points, pulmonary adducts were at least 6.9 times higher in the ELP group as compared with the IV group. Serum cisplatin levels were significantly higher after ELP, but there were no toxic pulmonary injuries in the ELP group. The authors concluded that this method resulted in greater DNA adduct formation than would be expected by simple dose escalation. In 2005, Jinbo and colleagues[20] established a technique for VATS ILP with cisplatin in a canine model and concluded that VATS–ILP provides a similar pharmacokinetic profile to conventional ILP. Matsuoka and colleagues[38] performed ILP with cisplatin in rats. When endothelin was injected in the PA before initiation of ILP, pulmonary toxicity was limited. Furthermore, significantly higher levels of total platinum were obtained in the tumors compared with normal lung tissue when compared with ILP alone.

COMPLICATIONS AND CONCERNS

As noted, multiple studies have shown that ILP is safe and reproducible. However, ILP remains an invasive procedure performed via a thoracotomy. ILP is limited to producing its effect during a single procedure, restricting clinical application when treating bulky or recurrent metastatic disease.[17]

Direct Lung Injury

The most obvious complication seen with ILP is injury to the lung itself. Franke and colleagues[19] examined the effects of varying mechanical parameters when performing ILP. They found a slight deterioration of all pulmonary function parameters compared with control animals with perfusion pressures higher than 25 mm Hg producing functional and morphologic damage to the perfused lung. Cisplatin ILP in rats revealed significant acute lung injury and compromised gas exchange function compared with the sham group.[18] Mild perivascular and peribronchial edema was noted with minimal hemorrhage and alveolar wall thickening for up to 21 days after ILP in canines.[20] In a similar manner, ILP has been shown to cause pulmonary hemorrhagic edema in pigs.[28] By comparison with the 30-minute standard perfusion, a gemcitabine ILP rat model study advised reducing perfusion to 6 minutes followed by delayed clamp release of no longer than 30 minutes to avoid reperfusion injury and acute respiratory distress syndrome.[30] This outcome highlighted the necessity to identify effective tissue saturation points relative to perfusion time to avoid unneeded risk.[30]

Results from human trials upheld the animal model results noted above. For example, during a phase I trial for melphalan 2 of 16 patients experienced grade 3 common toxicity criteria

(according to the National Cancer Institute) with lung edema and radiographic changes resembling chemical pneumonitis of the entire perfused lung.[12] In a phase I trial for doxorubicin, 1 of 8 patients developed significant chemical pneumonitis at 80 mg/m^2. In addition, all 7 patients perfused with 40 mg/m^2 experienced significant decrease in forced expiratory volume in 1 second and exhibited a trend toward decreased diffusing capacity.[10] In a phase I cisplatin ILP trial, pulmonary edema was a major complication that developed during feasibility trials when Ratto and colleagues[11] reported 2 of their 6 patients developing diffuse lung edema 48 hours after normothermic 200 mg/m^2 fixed dose cisplatin ILP performed over 60 minutes. One of these patients required respiratory support. In a 2002 study using hyperthemic 70 mg/m^2 fixed dose cisplatin ILP, no drug-related toxicity was observed but all patients developed noncardiogenic edema and ischemic mucosal changes in the treated lung and bronchial segments.[9]

Systemic Toxicity

Although ILP permits active drug agents to be administered at significantly higher doses compared with IV chemotherapy with minimal systemic effects, there remain acute and delayed pulmonary toxicities present in ILP treatment. One study found that transient vascular toxicity persists regardless of dosage when administering gemcitabine ILP in pigs. The research identified apparent capillary leak syndrome caused by gemcitabine itself, though no renal or hepatic toxicity was present.[35] Cisplatin ILP in rats noted that hyperthermia helped to alleviate the toxicity caused by cisplatin treatment; however, a dose-dependent damage of lung tissue trend was identified ($P<.001$; $R = 0.670$).[18] These results supported previous findings that cisplatin ILP was capable of high platinum concentrations of perfusate while producing poor systemic toxicity in rats and pigs.[5]

Phase I trials demonstrated mixed amounts of systemic leakage and toxicity. For instance, in a phase I trial for melphalan, 3 of the 7 patient groups at or below the MTD group reported 0.16 to 0.57 μg/mL systemic leakage after ILP.[12] In another example, 2 of 8 patients in a doxorubicin ILP phase I trial developed cardiac toxicity, which could not be fully evaluated owing to participant refusal or inability to tolerate the procedure.[10] Furthermore, a phase I TNF-α trial recorded 1 of the 20 patients exhibiting TNF toxicity (ie, decreased blood pressure, transient increase in creatinine, pulmonary insufficiency with bilateral infiltrates, and bronchorrhea) after a 10% leak rate during ILP.[13] Similarly, Hendriks and colleagues[5] recorded significant toxicity present at 15- and 45-mg doses during hyperthermia conditions.

Lung to Tumor Drug Concentration

With the importance of monitoring potential local and systemic toxicities while using cytotoxic agents, tumor to lung tissue drug concentration ratios should be maximized to decrease any damage to healthy tissue. Clearly, the advantage of ILP over IV treatment is improved locoregional delivery of cytotoxic agents while minimizing systemic effects. Conversely, several studies have noted significantly higher drug uptake in lung parenchyma compared with tumor tissue concentrations for both free and liposomal encapsulated doxorubicin ILP in high- and low-dose rat models.[22,23] Yan and colleagues[22] found 400 μg high-dose doxorubicin resulted in significantly higher tumor to lung drug concentration ratios (0.67 $\pm$ 0.2; P = .003) compared with 100 μg agent dose (0.27 $\pm$ 0.1; P = .003), contrasting findings that the same 100 to 400 μg increase in IV drug administration did not significantly improve the tumor to lung tissue ratio. Likewise, Cheng and colleagues[23] observed lung tissue uptake ratios significantly higher in normal tissue versus tumor tissue (13.8 $\pm$ 4.3 μg/g normal vs 3.9 $\pm$ 2.5 μg/g tumor, 100 μg dose) in rats.

Phase I cisplatin ILP produced lower or similar uptake in tumor tissue compared with lung tissue.[11] A doxorubicin ILP clinical trial had 3 of 4 patients report higher lung tissue uptake compared with tumor tissue drug uptake.[10] Unfortunately, other drugs trials have not yet produced definitive tumor to lung uptake ratios.

Heterogeneous Drug Distribution

Heterogeneous drug distribution patterns in normal lung parenchyma and tumor tissue after ILP has been observed in multiple animal models and for multiple cytotoxic drugs.[22,23,28,35] Pagès and colleges noted heterogeneous parenchymal concentrations of gemcitabine in pigs where the lower lobe parenchymal concentrations tended to be higher when higher doses were given. The study provided a possible explanation for the reported variations in gemcitabine concentration patterns via the nonsymmetrical branching inherent to bronchial and pulmonary vasculature in addition to capillary leak syndrome associated with gemcitabine itself. However, differences in sample localization complicated interpretation of the results.[35] In another study using rats, high-dose liposomal-encapsulated doxorubicin

increased drug concentration homogeneity.[22] Cheng and colleagues[23] reported lesser interanimal variability and spatial drug distribution in rat model IV treatments compared with doxorubicin and liposomal-encapsulated doxorubicin ILP.

SUMMARY

ILP is an investigational technique with a substantial body of literature to support its continued clinical application in patients who are not eligible for metasasectomy and its further development. ILP has been studied extensively in a variety of models including rats, dogs, pigs, sheep, and humans. In summation of these studies, ILP is a safe and reproducible technique that selectively delivers high doses of chemotherapeutic drugs to the lung with minimal frequency of the systemic toxic side effects commonly seen in IV chemotherapy. Current phase I clinical trials show that ILP can be safely performed in humans, but with mixed clinical results and poor long-term survival.

As noted in previous reviews, there is still a need for phase II and phase III clinical trials to determine the ultimate clinical utility of ILP. Although doxorubicin, FUDR, TNF-α, paclitaxel, melphalan, gemcitabine, and cisplatin are the most frequently studied chemotherapeutic agents, additional research into less investigated and novel single and combination drug therapies remain. New alternative techniques for ILP continue to be developed; however, significant improvements to patient outcomes remain as a goal for the future.

REFERENCES

1. Van Schil PE, Hendriks JM, Van Putte BP, et al. Isolated lung perfusion and related techniques for the treatment of pulmonary metastases. Eur J Cardiothorac Surg 2008;33(3):487–96.
2. Pastorino U, Buyse M, Friedel G, et al. Long-term results of lung metastasectomy: prognostic analyses based on 5206 cases. J Thorac Cardiovasc Surg 1997;113(1):37–49.
3. Rickaby DA, Fehring JF, Johnston MR, et al. Tolerance of the isolated perfused lung to hyperthermia. J Thorac Cardiovasc Surg 1991;101(4):732–9.
4. Cowen ME, Howard RB, Mulvin D, et al. Lung tolerance to hyperthermia by in vivo perfusion. Eur J Cardiothorac Surg 1992;6(4):167–72.
5. Hendriks JM, Van Putte BP, Grootenboers M, et al. Isolated lung perfusion for pulmonary metastases. Thorac Surg Clin 2006;16(2):185–98, vii.
6. Creech O, Krementz ET, Ryan RF, et al. Chemotherapy of cancer: regional perfusion utilizing an extracorporeal circuit. Ann Surg 1958;148(4):616–32.

7. Ranney DF. Drug targeting to the lungs. Biochem Pharmacol 1986;35(7):1063–9.

8. Johnston MR, Minchin R, Shull JH, et al. Isolated lung perfusion with adriamycin. A preclinical study. Cancer 1983;52:404–9.

9. Schröder C, Fisher S, Pieck AC, et al. Technique and results of hyperthermic (41 degrees C) isolated lung perfusion with high-doses of cisplatin for the treatment of surgically relapsing or unresectable lung sarcoma metastasis. Eur J Cardiothorac Surg 2002;22(1):41–6.

10. Burt ME, Liu D, Abolhoda A, et al. Isolated lung perfusion for patients with unresectable metastases from sarcoma: a phase I trial. Ann Thorac Surg 2000;69:1542–9.

11. Ratto GB, Toma S, Civalleri D, et al. Isolated lung perfusion with platinum in the treatment of pulmonary metastases from soft tissue sarcomas. J Thorac Cardiovasc Surg 1996;112(3):614–22.

12. Hendriks JM, Grootenboers MJ, Schramel FM, et al. Isolated lung perfusion with melphalan for resectable lung metastases: a phase I clinical trial. Ann Thorac Surg 2004;78(6):1919–26.

13. Pass HI, Mew DJ, Kranda KC, et al. Isolated lung perfusion with tumor necrosis factor for pulmonary metastases. Ann Thorac Surg 1996;61(6):1609–17.

14. Kümmerle A, Krueger T, Dusmet M, et al. A validated assay for measuring doxorubicin in biological fluids and tissues in an isolated lung perfusion model: matrix effect and heparin interference strongly influence doxorubicin measurements. J Pharm Biomed Anal 2003;33(3):475–94.

15. Schrump DS, Zhai S, Nguyen DM, et al. Pharmacokinetics of paclitaxel administered by hyperthermic retrograde isolated lung perfusion techniques. J Thorac Cardiovasc Surg 2002;123(4):686–94.

16. Furrer M, Lardinois D, Thormann W, et al. Cytostatic lung perfusion by use of an endovascular blood flow occlusion technique. Ann Thorac Surg 1998;65: 1523–8.

17. Van Putte BP, Hendriks JM, Romijn S, et al. Pharmacokinetics after pulmonary artery perfusion with gemcitabine. Ann Thorac Surg 2003;76(4):1036–40.

18. Franke UF, Wittwer T, Kaluza M, et al. Evaluation of isolated lung perfusion as neoadjuvant therapy of lung metastases using a novel in vivo pig model: II. High-dose cisplatin is well tolerated by the native lung tissue. Eur J Cardiothorac Surg 2004;26(4):800–6.

19. Franke UF, Wittwer T, Lessel M, et al. Evaluation of isolated lung perfusion as neoadjuvant therapy of lung metastases using a novel in vivo pig model: I. Influence of perfusion pressure and hyperthermia on functional and morphological lung integrity. Eur J Cardiothorac Surg 2004;26(4):792–9.

20. Jinbo M, Ueda K, Kaneda Y, et al. Video-assisted transcatheter lung perfusion regional chemotherapy. Eur J Cardiothorac Surg 2005;27(6):1079–82.

21. Baciewicz FA, Arredondo M, Chaudhuri B, et al. Pharmacokinetics and toxicity of isolated perfusion of lung with doxorubicin. J Surg Res 1991;50(2): 124–8.

22. Yan H, Cheng C, Haouala A, et al. Distribution of free and liposomal doxorubicin after isolated lung perfusion in a sarcoma model. Ann Thorac Surg 2008; 85(4):1225–32.

23. Cheng C, Haouala A, Krueger T, et al. Drug uptake in a rodent sarcoma model after intravenous injection or isolated lung perfusion of free/liposomal doxorubicin. Interact Cardiovasc Thorac Surg 2009;8(6):635–8.

24. Ng B, Lenert JT, Weksler B, et al. Isolated lung perfusion with FUDR is an effective treatment for colorectal adenocarcinoma lung metastases in rats. Ann Thorac Surg 1995;59(1):205–8.

25. Port JL, Ng B, Ellis JL, et al. Isolated lung perfusion with FUDR in the rat: pharmacokinetics and survival. Ann Thorac Surg 1996;62(3):848–52.

26. Nawata S, Abecasis N, Ross HM, et al. Isolated lung perfusion with melphalan for the treatment of metastatic pulmonary sarcoma. J Thorac Cardiovasc Surg 1996;112:1542–8.

27. Van Schil P, Hendriks J. Isolated lung perfusion for the treatment of pulmonary metastases an experimental study in the rat. Verh K Acad Geneeskd Belg 1999;61(4):517–50.

28. Van der Elst A, Oosterling SJ, Paul MA, et al. Isolated lung perfusion with melphalan: pharmacokinetics and toxicity in a pig model. J Surg Oncol 2006;93(5):410–6.

29. Van Putte BP, Hendriks JM, Romijn S, et al. Isolated lung perfusion with gemcitabine in a rat: pharmacokinetics and survival. J Surg Res 2003;109(2): 118–22.

30. Van Putte BP, Hendriks JM, Guetens G, et al. Modified approach of administering cytostatics to the lung: more efficient isolated lung perfusion. Ann Thorac Surg 2006;82(3):1033–7.

31. Van Putte BP, Grootenboers M, Van Boven WJ, et al. Pharmacokinetics of gemcitabine when delivered by selective pulmonary artery perfusion for the treatment of lung cancer. Drug Metab Dispos 2008; 36(4):676–81.

32. Grootenboers MJ, Schramel FM, Van Boven WJ, et al. Selective pulmonary artery perfusion followed by blood flow occlusion: new challenge for the treatment of pulmonary malignancies. Lung Cancer 2009;63(3):400–4.

33. Van Putte BP, Grootenboers M, Van Boven WJ, et al. Selective pulmonary artery perfusion for the treatment of primary lung cancer: improved drug exposure of the lung. Lung Cancer 2009;65(2): 208–13.

34. Pagès PB, Facy O, Mordant P, et al. Isolated lung perfusion as an adjuvant treatment of colorectal

cancer lung metastases: a preclinical study in a pig model. PLoS One 2013;8(3):e59485.

35. Pagès PB, Derangere V, Bouchot O, et al. Acute and delayed toxicity of gemcitabine administered during isolated lung perfusion: a preclinical dose-escalation study in pigs. Eur J Cardiothorac Surg 2015;48(2):228–35.

36. Saeki K, Kaneda Y, Li TS, et al. Relationship between the concentration of CDDP in tumor and tumor size after isolated lung perfusion treatment experimental

study on a solitary pulmonary sarcoma model in rats. J Surg Oncol 2000;75(3):193–6.

37. Brown DB, Ma MK, Battafarano RJ, et al. Endovascular lung perfusion using high-dose cisplatin: uptake and DNA adduct formation in an animal model. Oncol Rep 2004;11(1):237–43.

38. Matsuoka T, Kaneda Y, Li TS, et al. Increasing drug concentration in a rat lung tumor model by combining isolated lung perfusion with hypertensive chemotherapy. Anticancer Res 2001;21(2A):1219–23.

Immunotherapy for Resected Pulmonary Metastases

Michael A. Morse, MD, MHS

KEYWORDS

• TIL • IL-2 • Interferon • Anti-PD-1 • Anti-PD-L1 • Cancer vaccine

KEY POINTS

- It is hypothesized that adjuvant immunotherapy may reduce the risk of recurrence of malignancies following resection of lung metastases.
- Adjuvant immunotherapy tested in melanoma and renal cell carcinoma includes tumor-infiltrating lymphocytes; cancer vaccines; cytokines, such as interleukin 2 and interferon; and checkpoint blockade molecules.
- Adjuvant immunotherapy tested in sarcomas have included interferon, liposomal muramyl-tripeptide-phosphatidylethanolamine, chimeric antigen receptor T cells, and cancer vaccines.
- Adjuvant immunotherapies tested in colorectal cancer have included tumor cell and dendritic cell–based vaccines.

BACKGROUND ON IMMUNE SYSTEM AND IMMUNOTHERAPY/IMMUNITY IN THE LUNG

The high rate of recurrence after metastasectomy of most malignancies demonstrates that controlling micrometastatic disease remains a challenge. Although there has been considerable interest in applying chemotherapy and targeted therapies to prevent recurrence, Immunotherapy has appeal, as by its very nature the immune system has both innate and adaptive elements that could provide long-term control of tumors, prevention of new tumors, and, potentially, elimination of the more aggressive clones, all possible with limited cycles of therapy. Furthermore, it is clear from most animal models of immunotherapy that immune effectors are most effective against the smallest volumes of disease, such that adjuvant therapy may have the greatest potential to demonstrate efficacy of immunotherapy.

Immunotherapy takes advantage of or interacts with the processes that lead to activation of immune responses naturally.[1] Tumor-specific immune responses depend on the uptake of tumor proteins, peptides, and genetic material (antigens) released during cell death by professional antigen-presenting cells (dendritic cells), which process and present the tumor antigens to T cells along with costimulatory molecules, which leads to T-cell activation and indirectly B-cell activation.

It is well established that T cells and antibodies that recognize tumors (T cells through T-cell receptor [TCR] recognition of their cognate peptide presented within major histocompatibility complex [MHC] class I or II molecules on the tumor surface and antibodies by binding to 3-dimensional structures recognized by their complementarity determining regions) are present in the tumor-bearing host and can have antitumor activity. T-cell activation can also be countered by upregulated expression of inhibitory molecules (eg, CTLA4).[2] Activated T cells traffic to and infiltrate the tumor. Those that are not suppressed by regulatory T cells and

Disclosure statement: Dr M.A. Morse has received honoraria from Prometheus.
Division of Medical Oncology, Duke University Medical Center, MSRB Room 403, Box 3233, Research Drive, Durham, NC 27710, USA
E-mail address: mihael.morse@duke.edu

Thorac Surg Clin 26 (2016) 69–78
http://dx.doi.org/10.1016/j.thorsurg.2015.09.009

myeloid-derived suppressor cells and their cyto-kines have the opportunity to bind to tumor cells expressing their cognate antigen and set off a cascade of events culminating in tumor cell death; however, some T cells that express the activation marker programmed death-1 (PD-1)[3] are suppressed by tumor-expressed PD ligand-1 (PD-L1). T-cell destruction of tumor releases antigens that can begin the cycle again if they are taken up by dendritic cells. Therefore, immunotherapies may be applied at all key steps in the immunity cycle, the initial phase of antigen delivery to dendritic cells (vaccines), T-cell activation (cytokines), trafficking of T cells to tumor (chemokines), and then T-cell attack on tumor cells recognized by the TCR (tumor-infiltrating lymphocytes [TILs] and chimeric antigen-receptor T cells [CAR-Ts]), and preservation of T-cell functionality (anti-PD-1 and anti-PD-L1 antibodies). Because metastasectomy provides fresh tumor tissue, it is particularly suited to strategies that use tumor-derived components as part of the immunotherapy strategy. For example, TILs may be retrieved from disaggregated tissue and cultured in vitro before re-administration as adoptive immunotherapy. Although TILs may be functionally suppressed in the tumor milieu, when cultured ex vivo in interleukin 2 (IL-2), their functionality as demonstrated by expression of TCR zeta and epsilon chains, p56, FAS, and FAS-ligand is increased. Other tumor constituents, including the malignant cells themselves and peptide, protein, and mRNA derivatives, may be used as components in cancer vaccines.

Although the lungs have a different immune milieu by virtue of the exposure to a panoply of air-borne allergens compared with the bowel or liver that are exposed to orally administered antigens or the skin that is exposed to contact immunogens and the different microbiome, there are limited data on whether considerations for immunotherapy for resected pulmonary metastases should be different than that of immunotherapy for resected liver metastases, for example. Therefore, this review attempts to focus on issues relevant for pulmonary metastasectomy but also discusses immunotherapy for other sights of metastases where relevant. What may differ is the immune response, in particular the T-cell infiltration into tumor, for different malignancies. For example, Rosenberg's group at the National Cancer Institute observed that fewer CD3+ T cells were found to infiltrate gastrointestinal (GI) cancer compared with melanoma metastases (to liver and lungs) and very few TILs from GI cancer metastases were tumor reactive.[4] Therefore, the author discusses immunotherapy considerations for different tumors separately.

MELANOMA

It is well established that the immune system responds to melanoma and it is in melanoma that many of the established tumor antigens were first identified and new discoveries on targeting tumor antigens are being made.[5] Higher total and CD8+ T-cell frequency in melanoma metastases is associated with improved overall survival (OS),[6] and numerous immunologic approaches have demonstrated antitumor activity for unresectable metastatic disease.[7] Immunotherapy with interferon-α (IFN-α) and its pegylated form[8] have long been a standard adjuvant therapy based on the recurrence-free survival (RFS) and OS benefit in resected stage III melanoma. IFNs have direct antitumor activity and are involved in activation of T and B cells, macrophages, and natural killer (NK) cells. More recently, the anti-CTLA4 antibody ipilimumab improved recurrence-free survival compared with placebo in resected stage III melanoma.[9] Tested in a randomized study following resection of stage IIIB/IIIC/IV or mucosal melanoma, recombinant granulocyte-macrophage colony-stimulating factor (GM-CSF) showed an improvement in disease-free survival (DFS) and a trend toward improved OS in the subgroup of patients with stage IV disease compared with placebo.[10] These data support the hypothesis that immunotherapy could have a role in resected metastatic melanoma, including pulmonary metastasectomies.

Although none were focused on pulmonary metastases, several studies have evaluated patients who have undergone lymphadenectomy or metastasectomy to determine whether various immunotherapies might reduce recurrence. Single-arm studies of vaccines following metastasectomies, in aggregate, have demonstrated long-term survival, although the number with lung metastasectomies is small.[11] Unfortunately, a phase III randomized protocol comparing polyvalent-cultured melanoma cell vaccine (Canvaxin) combined with BCG versus BCG alone for patients with resected stage III/IV melanoma was closed early for futility due to failure to improve DFS and OS and a decrease in survival for vaccinated patients.[12] A single-arm study of patients with stage III/IV melanoma (the majority with macroscopic lymph node metastases but some with resected stage IV disease) who had no evidence of disease after surgery tested dendritic cells (DC) electroporated with mRNA encoding a fusion protein between MAGE-A1, -A3, -C2; tyrosinase; MelanA/MART-1; or gp100 and an HLA class II–targeting sequence along with IFN-α-2b.[13] The median OS had not been reached; the 2-year and 4-year survival rates were 93% and 70%, respectively. Although the lack of a control group does not allow direct assessment of the impact of the vaccine, comparison with similar patients treated with IFN alone suggested a favorable survival benefit. Further, the investigators commented that some recurrences were single lesions that could be resected leading again to no evidence of disease. Whether immunotherapy is associated with more indolent recurrences or whether patients who can undergo metastasectomy have tumor biology more likely to lead to limited recurrences is unclear.

As noted earlier, because metastasectomy provides access to tumor tissue from which TILs may be extracted and activated, it is well suited to applications using TILs. Although TIL therapy has been predominantly reported in the setting of advanced metastatic disease, there is some reported experience following metastasectomy to prevent recurrence. The potentially greater efficacy of TILs in patients after metastasectomy compared with active metastatic disease was suggested by a preliminary study of adoptive TIL in combination with IL-2 in patients with advanced melanoma, colorectal carcinoma, and renal cell carcinoma, which was followed by enrollment of patients with no evidence of disease following metastasectomy.[14] Although there was no objective response observed in the advanced patients and all progressed after a median of 1.5 months, among the adjuvant postmetastasectomy patients, more than half (13 of 22) remained disease free after a median of 23+ months. Follow-up data from these patients demonstrated that 64.7% (11 of 17) of the initially disease-free group were still free of disease after a median of 37+ months (range, 5+ - 69+).[15] In a follow-up single-arm study of TIL administered with infusions of IL-2 to patients with stage III/IV melanoma who underwent resection of metachronous metastases,[16] a total of 8 of 22 (36.3%) evaluable patients were disease free at a median follow-up of 5 years. Again, it is difficult to determine whether these results exceed those of other modalities but does provide additional feasibility and long-term safety data that could support randomized studies in the future.

Based on activity for systemically administered, high-dose IL-2 against metastatic melanoma and the widespread experience with inhalation therapies, both inhaled low-dose[17] and high-dose[18] IL-2 have been studied. Although not a postmetastasectomy study, the high-dose IL-2 experience[18] is instructive of several issues regarding effects of the therapy. Patients with pulmonary-predominant metastatic melanoma received dacarbazine (DTIC) and inhalation IL-2 therapy (36 million IU

per day, 6 days per week, monthly). Demonstrating the local rather than regional activity of this strategy was the observation that there were no responses to treatment outside of the lung; but for lung metastases, there were 18.5% durable complete response (CR) (5 of 27), 29.6% (8 of 27) partial response (PR), and 18.5% (5 of 27) stable disease (SD), rates higher than expected from DTIC alone. Most of the SD and PR progressed (off therapy) by 6 months, suggesting the need for continued therapy. Mild fever and cough were the predominant toxicities, dramatically lower than intravenous high-dose IL-2 regimens. There were no correlative studies evaluating the intrapulmonary immune response, so the mechanism of activity is speculative. The lower-dose study[17] enrolled previously treated patients with lung metastatic melanoma and patients who had undergone pulmonary metastasectomy, receiving IL-2 as prophylaxis against recurrence. All received daily inhalations of 3×3 million IU recombinant IL-2 on an ongoing basis. Patients with extrapulmonary metastases also received DTIC intravenously. Clinical benefit included PR (27%) or SD (33%) but no CR in those with metastatic disease. Those with clinical benefit tended to develop few new pulmonary metastases subsequently. None of the postmetastasectomy patients showed recurrence of lung metastases during the treatment period (median 24.5 months). The investigators noted their lack of CR compared with the high-dose experience, which did report CR. They think this is related to the fact that most patients in the low-dose study had extrapulmonary metastases compared with half in the high-dose study.

Another concern with this approach is that in pulmonary metastasectomy patients, the most common site of subsequent recurrence is an extrapulmonary visceral organ (44% in one study[19]), suggesting systemic therapy could still be needed along with inhalation therapy. GM-CSF that stimulates dendritic cells leading to enhanced immune responses has also been studied for inhalation therapy in patients with advanced melanoma, demonstrating safety and activation systemic immune responses in a minority of patients; but clinical efficacy data are limited.[20]

As anti–PD-1 and anti–PD-L1 have demonstrated significant activity in metastatic melanoma,[21] there is of course interest in their efficacy in the adjuvant setting. Gibney[22] treated HLA-A*0201–positive patients with the anti–PD-1 antibody nivolumab (1 mg/kg, 3 mg/kg, or 10 mg/kg intravenously) with a multi-peptide vaccine (gp100, MART-1, and NY-ESO-1 with Montanide ISA 51 VG) every 2 weeks for 12 doses followed by nivolumab maintenance every 12 weeks for 8 doses. Of the 31 patients with metastases, 7 had lung metastasis resected. Overall, 10 of 33 patients relapsed; the median relapse-free survival (RFS) was 47.1 months. Given the tolerability and efficacy of PD-1/PD-L1 targeting therapy, it is likely that it will be tested as an adjuvant more commonly in the future.

Although most of the studies using immunotherapy and surgery report immunotherapy as a postoperative adjuvant, it is also possible to administer immunotherapy and then resect residual disease. Reasons for residual disease could include tumor antigenic heterogeneity with some masses not expressing antigens recognizable by T cells or downregulation of MHC molecules by tumors or failure of T cells to infiltrate these tumors. Removing these resistant sites would allow elimination of the disease. Yang and colleagues[23] reported that among patients with melanoma with partial responses to high-dose IL-2, surgical salvage results in approximately 20% of patients seeming to be cured and 36% surviving for at least 5 years after salvage surgery.

In summary, because pulmonary metastasectomy of melanoma is associated with longer survival but a significant risk of extrapulmonary visceral relapse, adjuvant systemic therapies (or local plus systemic therapies) will likely be necessary. The availability of the tumor provides an opportunity for TIL therapy, and the demonstrated efficacy of systemic immunotherapies in melanoma in general provides additional tools for combination to enhance the survival rate.

RENAL CELL CARCINOMA

Renal cell carcinoma (RCC) is frequently lymphocyte infiltrated, suggesting it is a target for immune effectors; however, immune dysfunction arises from both defective dendritic cell differentiation and anergy-associated genes in T cells.[24] An important observation in RCC is that removing the primary tumor before immunotherapy enhances the survival benefit from the immunotherapy.[25,26] The explanation for this observation is still debated, but it is assumed that the primary tumor harbors cytokines (IL-4, IL-10, transforming growth factor-β [TGF-β], vascular endothelial growth factor) or cell types (T regulatory cells [Treg], myeloid derived suppressor cell [MDSC]) that cause dendritic cell or T-cell dysfunction. Lauerova[27] reported that reduced CD80+ and CD19+/80+ cells (presumably antigen-presenting cells expressing costimulatory molecules) before nephrectomy was associated with a greater risk of relapse after IL-2/IFN immunotherapy; however, Wald[28] found that early after

nephrectomy, there was little change in the peripheral blood immune parameters except for a decrease in the CD8+ T cells expressing the inhibitory molecule B- and T-lymphocyte attenuator (BTLA). There are no data regarding changes in the immune milieu of the metastatic sites following nephrectomy. Further, it is not known how the resection of the metastases may alter immune responses to micrometastatic disease. Nonetheless, the data regarding improved outcome of immunotherapy after nephrectomy support the hypothesis that removing metastases could alter immune function and enhance the efficacy of postmetastasectomy immunotherapy.

The role of adjuvant immunotherapy for RCC, localized or metastatic, remains unclear. In a study of adjuvant DC vaccination combined with cytokine-induced killer cell therapy after RCC resection,[29] there was a prolonged PFS and reduced mortality compared with patients receiving IFN. In a randomized study of autologous tumor lysate-pulsed DCs and cytokine-induced killer cells compared with IFN-α or no postoperative adjuvant therapy for resected localized or locally advanced RCC,[30] OS was significantly greater in the DC/cytokine-induced killer group and IFN-α group than that in the control group; but there was no difference between the DC/cytokine-induced killer group and IFN-α group. Unfortunately, studies of adjuvant autologous tumor cells or cytokines after resection of primary tumors have not demonstrated survival benefits.[31–33] Similarly, a nonrandomized trial comparing patients who received immunotherapy after metastasectomy of RCC also concluded that there was no difference in survival for those who received postoperative immunotherapy.[34]

Newer agents under development, such as anti-CTLA4 antibodies and PD-1/PD-L1 antibodies, have demonstrated preliminary evidence of activity in metastatic RCC.[35,36] For example, response rates ranged from 43% to 48% with nivolumab/ipilimumab and 52% with nivolumab/sunitinib. Whether there is enough of a T-cell infiltrate in micrometastatic disease to benefit from blockade of T-cell inhibitory pathways is unclear, but these high response rates support use as adjuvant therapy. Achieving a T-cell infiltrate may require use of cancer vaccines. Vaccines based on peptides and viral vectors and dendritic cell vaccines that have been tested or are in late-phase studies in RCC include IMA901, TG-4010, MVA-5T4,[37,38] and the personalized DC-based therapy AGS-003.[39–41] Preliminary data with AGS-003 indicate improved PFS and OS when compared with historic controls of patients with unfavorable-risk metastatic renal cell carcinoma (mRCC). Again, these have not been tested after metastasectomy but would be theoretically applicable because autologous tissue would be available from this procedure.

As with melanoma, inhaled IL-2 has been administered for pulmonary metastases of IL-2 (although not as adjuvant therapy).[42] Interestingly, there was a suggestion that the inhaled IL-2 could be associated with a greater chance of long-term survival than systemic IL-2.

SARCOMA

Sarcoma was one of the first areas where observations on immunotherapy of cancer were made.[43] The lymphocytic response to sarcomas has been studied to a limited degree and seems to be more complicated to characterize than in other malignancies. CD3+, CD4+, and CD8+ T-cell infiltration did not correlate with outcomes; but intratumoral CD20+ B-cell density was a good prognosis factor in patients with wide resection margins. However, in another study from this group, a high density of CD20+ lymphocytes in the peritumoral capsule was a negative prognostic indicator, and there was no effect on prognosis of CD20 counts in tumor.[44,45] They did not study pulmonary metastases. Coexpression of M-CSF and TGF-β in tumor was independent from negative prognostic factors for disease-specific survival.[46] The role of PD-L1/PD-1 axis is also not clear for sarcomas. In a pathology study of various sarcomas,[47] lymphocyte and macrophage infiltration was present in 98% and 90%, respectively; tumor, lymphocyte, and macrophage PD-L1 expression was noted in 12%, 30%, and 58%, respectively, with the highest prevalence in GI stromal tumors (29%). There was no association between clinical features, OS, and PD-L1 expression in tumor or immune infiltrates. This finding suggests that there could be other factors affecting the immune response to sarcoma; however, sarcomas are immunogenic in preclinical models and express well-recognized tumor antigens, including cancer testis antigens (NY-ESO-1, LAGE, PRAME, MAGE-A3) and gangliosides (GM2, disialoganglioside [GD2], and GD3), with expression varying by histologic subtype.[48]

Immunotherapy of sarcomas was recently reviewed.[48] IFNs that have both direct antitumor activity and are involved in T and B cells, macrophages, and NK-cell activation have been tested as adjuvants for resected sarcoma.[49] Initial series suggested long-term survival benefit was possible for patients with osteosarcoma treated adjuvantly with IFN-containing regimens but subsequent study did not.[50–52] The more recent EURAMOS-1 (NCT00134030) study randomized patients with osteosarcoma with a good response (<10% viable tumor at surgery) to induction chemotherapy, 4 cycles of chemotherapy with and without maintenance pegylated IFN-α-2b.[53] Although the hazard ratio for event-free survival (EFS) from the adjusted Cox model was 0.82 in favor of MAP plus IFN, it was not statistically significant. None of these studies directly studied resected lung metastases.

Liposomal muramyl-tripeptide-phosphatidylethanolamine (L-MTP-PE; mifamurtide), an inflammation-inducing synthetic bacterial cell wall analogue incorporated into liposomes to target delivery to monocytes and macrophages in areas such as the lungs, was tested in the Children's Oncology Group Intergroup-0133 study in which patients with osteosarcoma without clinically detectable metastatic disease were randomized to one of 2 chemotherapy combinations and then to receive or not receive MTP. EFS and OS were increased in those who received chemotherapy with L-MTP-PE (5-year OS: 78% vs 70%).[54] Subsequent analysis[55] of the group with metastases (including lung metastases) did not show a significant EFS and OS, but the investigators concluded that there was a trend for improved survival for patients receiving L-MTP-PE. In a nonrandomized study of patients with high-risk, recurrent, and/or metastatic osteosarcoma,[56] L-MTP-PE with and without chemotherapy was associated with survival comparable with prior studies with this agent and 2-year OS of 45.9%; but the nonrandomized nature of the study precluded more definitive conclusions.

Multiple small studies have reported on cancer vaccines for patients with sarcomas[48]; a randomized phase II trial of a vaccine intended to activate antibody responses against the gangliosides GD2, GD3, and GM2 is being studied in patients who have undergone metastasectomy (NCT01141491); but the results are unavailable. A recent study of autologous tumor vaccines modified to secrete GM-CSF[57] in patients with advanced alveolar soft-part sarcoma and clear cell sarcoma (chosen because they have some biological similarities to melanoma) demonstrated immunogenicity but no tumor regression. However, tumor biopsies showed PD-1–positive CD8+ T cells located in association with PD-L1–expressing sarcoma cells. This finding suggests the potential role of PD-1/PD-L1 targeting therapies.

Because established tumor antigens have been identified as expressed by sarcomas, adoptive cell transfer with TILS, T cells modified to express tumor antigen-specific TCRs,[58] or CAR-Ts (T cells modified to express chimeric antigen receptor for a tumor antigen, often in conjunction with additional components of T-cell signaling) have been studied. A recent report suggested the possible utility of this approach.[59] The investigators generated IGF1R and ROR1 CAR-Ts based on observation of IGF1R and ROR1 expression in most Ewing sarcoma, osteosarcoma, alveolar or embryonal rhabdomyosarcoma, and fibrosarcoma cell lines. Adoptive transfer of the IGF1R and ROR1 CAR-Ts derived from a patient with sarcoma significantly reduced tumor growth in osteosarcoma xenograft models. In a phase I/II clinical trial of 19 patients with recurrent/refractory HER2-positive tumors (16 osteosarcomas, one Ewing sarcoma, one primitive neuroectodermal tumor, and one desmoplastic small round cell tumor)[60] received HER2–CAR-Ts. The T-cell infusions were well tolerated without dose-limiting toxicity, and 4 of 17 evaluable patients had stable disease for 12 weeks to 14 months. The median OS was 10.3 months (range, 5.1–29.1 months). A patient with osteosarcoma who had lung/pleural metastases resected after T-cell infusions was noted to have experienced 90% or greater necrosis of the tumor. The HER2–CAR-Ts persisted for at least 6 weeks in most receiving the highest doses; importantly, HER2–CAR-Ts could traffic to tumors as they were detected at tumor sites of 2 of 2 patients examined; however, there are limited data as to whether CAR-Ts can traffic to micrometastatic disease. Therefore, it is unclear whether CAR-Ts will eventually be used as adjuvant therapy after metastasectomy of sarcoma.

COLON CANCER

T-cell infiltration into colorectal cancers is associated with improved survival in those with resected disease (although the association is less clear for metastases).[61] Further, the induction of an immune response by cancer vaccines has been associated with a clinical benefit.[62,63] Prior studies of vaccination following liver metastasectomy of colon cancer have suggested clinical benefits in subgroup analyses.[64–67] A study comparing 2 dendritic cell vaccine strategies[67] following resection of metastases enrolled 26 patients with liver (n = 24) and lung (n = 2) metastases. Among the 24 who were disease free at the time of vaccination, the RFS was 58% at 1 year, 42% at 2 years, and 38% at 5 years. After more than 5 years of follow-up, 8 are alive and disease free, 4 are alive with recurrent disease, and 12 have died of colorectal cancer. RFS was higher for the 11 patients who developed a tumor-specific immune response following vaccination. Because there was no significant difference in RFS between the patients who had evidence of

an immune response against a control antigen and those with no immune response and patients with no evidence of response, this was thought to be the result of an induction against tumor antigen rather than a better outcome merely because of better immune biology. The author's group reported adjuvant treatment of patients with colorectal cancer with a DC vaccine after metastasis resection. In this study, 9 of 13 patients treated with a carcinoembryonic antigen (CEA) mRNA-loaded DC vaccine relapsed at a median of 122 days, and few antipeptide responses were detected.[68] More recently, the author performed a phase II randomized clinical trial[69] comparing autologous DC modified with poxvectors encoding CEA and MUC1 and costimulatory molecules (CD54, CD58, CD80) versus the poxvectors alone in 76 patients who had undergone resection of hepatic or pulmonary metastases. Approximately 25% in each arm had lung metastases. The RFS was similar for both arms and a contemporary control group, but the OS was longer for the combined group of vaccinated patients compared with the control group. The author did not separate the results by the presence of lung or liver metastases. Survival was longer for patients who developed an immune response to the vaccine-encoded CEA.

The author has also studied premetastasectomy Flt3 ligand (FLT3L) administration.[70] FLT3L is a cytokine that stimulates bone marrow progenitors, increases DC in the peripheral blood and tumor, and heightens T-cell responses and NK function, resulting in antitumor activity.[71] Of the 12 patients enrolled, 7 patients had liver metastases and 5 had lung metastases. As expected, the percentage of CD11c(+)CD14(−) DCs in peripheral blood mononuclear cells PBMCs increased. Although there were no objective responses, there was an increase in the number of DCs observed at the periphery of the tumors of patients who received FLT3L compared with those of patients who had not. One patient with multiple pulmonary metastases who underwent resection, then received FLT3L followed by another resection, had an increase (nearly two-fold) in the number of fascin-positive DCs in the second specimen. Another patient who received FLT3L followed by a pulmonary metastasis resection and then another cycle of FLT3L followed by a second resection had a three-fold increase in the number of fascin-positive DC in the periphery of the tumor from the second specimen. Further, delayed-type hypersensitivity responses to recall antigens (candida, mumps, and tetanus) showed marginally significant increases in reactivity after FLT3L administration. These data suggested that pretreatment cytokines could induce an immune response directed at the tumor with the hope that this response may persist after surgery. With a median follow-up of 300 days, 6 of the 8 patients who underwent resections had recurrences at a median period of 256 days; but long-term survival data are not available.

In summary, there may be a benefit for adjuvant therapy after metastasectomy of colorectal cancer but larger, randomized studies will be required. Further, subgroups with particularly high responses to immunotherapy may be the preferred group. For example, colorectal cancers with mismatch repair (MMR) defects (microsatellite instability high) are highly T-cell infiltrated.[72] Le and colleagues[73] recently reported that patients with MMR-deficient colon cancer experienced response rates and disease control rates of 40% and 90% following pembrolizumab administration. These exciting results open the possibility of using adjuvant immunotherapy in this small, but important, subgroup.

OTHER MALIGNANCIES

Pulmonary metastasectomy is occasional performed for other malignancies, which have been studied as targets for immunotherapy. For example, lung cancers presenting with metachronous metastases to the lung may be candidates for a resection. Immunotherapy of lung cancer has been an area of significant interest, but studies of adjuvant vaccination have not been successful. For example, in the highly anticipated MAGRIT trial,[74] a randomized trial of recombinant MAGE-3 plus AS15 adjuvant versus placebo for completely resected (R0), MAGE-A3–positive non–small cell lung cancer (stages IB, II, and IIIA) following standard therapy, there was no improvement in DFS with the vaccine. The recent reports of efficacy for the anti–PD-1 targeting therapy[75] for non–small cell lung cancer opens the possibility for ultimately using these drugs as adjuvant therapies.

Breast cancer has also been the focus of numerous immunotherapy studies. In phase I/II clinical trials in which patients with breast cancer were vaccinated with E75 (nelipepimut-S) HER2 peptide and GM-CSF in the adjuvant setting,[76] the 5-year DFS was 89.7% in the vaccinated patients versus 80.2% in the control group. Although this was not statistically significant, among patients who were optimally doses, there was a statistically significant reduction in recurrence. These data support possible immunotherapy studies following resection of lung metastases of breast cancer.

Bladder cancer, at least the localized form, has been treated with immunologic therapies, such as BCG installation[77]; but such therapy is unlikely to be applicable for resected metastases. However, the recent demonstration of benefit for anti–PD-L1 therapy[78] in advanced urothelial cancers also raises the question of whether it could be used as an adjuvant in the future.

SUMMARY

Adjuvant immunotherapy has been of substantial interest because of the hope of preventing recurrences after surgical resection of primary or metastatic disease without the toxic chemotherapies that are currently used. Although lung metastases could present a biologically different immune milieu, adjuvant immunotherapy studies have, in general, not focused on pulmonary metastasectomies; therefore, immunotherapies that are in development for disease at any site of the body are likely reasonable candidates to test in patients who have undergone pulmonary metastasectomies. The availability of tumor tissue has fueled enthusiasm for vaccines based on tumor cells or their constituents and for T-cell therapeutics based on the TILs extracted from tumor tissue. The high rates of clinical activity in some malignancies following anti–PD-1 or anti–PD-L1 therapy has now suggested these biologics may be tested as adjuvant therapies following surgical resections. More efficacious therapies may of course increase the number who may undergo metastasectomies, and debulking metastasectomies may become of greater interest if it is known that adjuvant therapies may be able to control the growth of small-volume residual disease.

REFERENCES

1. Giraldo NA, Becht E, Vano Y, et al. The immune response in cancer: from immunology to pathology to immunotherapy. Virchows Arch 2015;467(2): 127–35.
2. Schneider H, Rudd CE. Diverse mechanisms regulate the surface expression of immunotherapeutic target ctla-4. Front Immunol 2014;5:619.
3. Boussiotis VA, Chatterjee P, Li L. Biochemical signaling of PD-1 on T cells and its functional implications. Cancer J 2014;20(4):265–71.
4. Turcotte S, Gros A, Hogan K, et al. Phenotype and function of T cells infiltrating visceral metastases from gastrointestinal cancers and melanoma: implications for adoptive cell transfer therapy. J Immunol 2013;191(5):2217–25.

5. Andrews MC, Woods K, Cebon J, et al. Evolving role of tumor antigens for future melanoma therapies. Future Oncol 2014;10(8):1457–68.

6. Kluger HM, Zito CR, Barr ML, et al. Characterization of PD-L1 expression and associated T-cell infiltrates in metastatic melanoma samples from variable anatomic sites. Clin Cancer Res 2015;21(13):3052–60.

7. Johnson DB, Sosman JA. Therapeutic advances and treatment options in metastatic melanoma. JAMA Oncol 2015;1(3):380–6.

8. Di Trolio R, Simeone E, Di Lorenzo G, et al. The use of interferon in melanoma patients: a systematic review. Cytokine Growth Factor Rev 2015; 26(2):203–12.

9. Eggermont AM, Chiarion-Sileni V, Grob JJ, et al. Adjuvant ipilimumab versus placebo after complete resection of high-risk stage III melanoma (EORTC 18071): a randomised, double-blind, phase 3 trial. Lancet Oncol 2015;16(5):522–30.

10. Lawson DH, Lee SJ, Tarhini AA, et al. E4697: phase III cooperative group study of yeast-derived granulocyte macrophage colony stimulating factor (GM-CSF) versus placebo as adjuvant treatment of patients with completely resected stage III-IV melanoma. J Clin Oncol 2010;28 [abstr: 8504].

11. Tagawa ST, Cheung E, Banta W, et al. Survival analysis after resection of metastatic disease followed by peptide vaccines in patients with stage IV melanoma. Cancer 2006;106(6):1353–7.

12. Morton DL, Mozzillo N, Thompson JF, et al, Malignant Melanoma Active Immunotherapy Trial 3 (MMAIT) Investigators. An international, randomized, phase III trial of bacillus Calmette-Guerin (BCG) plus allogeneic melanoma vaccine (MCV) or placebo after complete resection of melanoma metastatic to regional or distant sites. J Clin Oncol 2007; 25(18S[June 20 supplement]):8508.

13. Wilgenhof S, Corthals J, Van Nuffel AM, et al. Long-term clinical outcome of melanoma patients treated with messenger RNA-electroporated dendritic cell therapy following complete resection of metastases. Cancer Immunol Immunother 2015;64(3): 381–8.

14. Ridolfi R, Flamini E, Riccobon A, et al. Adjuvant adoptive immunotherapy with tumour-infiltrating lymphocytes and modulated doses of interleukin-2 in 22 patients with melanoma, colorectal and renal cancer, after radical metastasectomy, and in 12 advanced patients. Cancer Immunol Immunother 1998;46(4):185–93.

15. Fabbri M, Ridolfi R, Maltoni R, et al. Tumor infiltrating lymphocytes and continuous infusion interleukin-2 after metastasectomy in 61 patients with melanoma, colorectal and renal carcinoma. Tumori 2000;86(1): 46–52.

16. Ridolfi L, Ridolfi R, Riccobon A, et al. Adjuvant immunotherapy with tumor infiltrating lymphocytes and interleukin-2 in patients with resected stage III and IV melanoma. J Immunother 2003;26(2):156–62.

17. Posch C, Weihsengruber F, Bartsch K, et al. Low-dose inhalation of interleukin-2 bio-chemotherapy for the treatment of pulmonary metastases in melanoma patients. Br J Cancer 2014;110(6): 1427–32.

18. Enk AH, Nashan D, Rübben A, et al. High dose inhalation interleukin-2 therapy for lung metastases in patients with malignant melanoma. Cancer 2000; 88(9):2042–6.

19. Neuman HB, Patel A, Hanlon C, et al. Stage-IV melanoma and pulmonary metastases: factors predictive of survival. Ann Surg Oncol 2007;14(10): 2847–53.

20. Markovic SN, Suman VJ, Nevala WK, et al. A dose-escalation study of aerosolized sargramostim in the treatment of metastatic melanoma: an NCCTG Study. Am J Clin Oncol 2008;31(6):573–9.

21. Mahoney KM, Freeman GJ, McDermott DF. The next immune-checkpoint inhibitors: PD-1/PD-L1 blockade in melanoma. Clin Ther 2015;37(4):764–82.

22. Gibney GT, Kudchadkar RR, DeConti RC, et al. Safety, correlative markers, and clinical results of adjuvant nivolumab in combination with vaccine in resected high-risk metastatic melanoma. Clin Cancer Res 2015;21(4):712–20.

23. Yang JC, Abad J, Sherry R. Treatment of oligometastases after successful immunotherapy. Semin Radiat Oncol 2006;16(2):131–5.

24. Noessner E, Brech D, Mendler AN, et al. Intratumoral alterations of dendritic-cell differentiation and CD8(+) T-cell anergy are immune escape mechanisms of clear cell renal cell carcinoma. Oncoimmunology 2012;1(8):1451–3.

25. Flanigan RC, Mickisch G, Sylvester R, et al. Cytoreductive nephrectomy in patients with metastatic renal cancer: a combined analysis. J Urol 2004; 171:1071–6.

26. Mickisch GH, Garin A, Van Poppel H, et al. Radical nephrectomy plus interferon-alfa-based immunotherapy compared with interferon alfa alone in metastatic renal-cell carcinoma: a randomized trial. Lancet 2001;358:966–70.

27. Lauerová L, Dusek L, Spurny V, et al. Relation of pre-nephrectomy CD profiles and serum cytokines to the disease outcome and response to IFN-alpha/IL-2 therapy in renal cell carcinoma patients. Oncol Rep 2001;8(3):685–92.

28. Wald G, Barnes KT, Bing MT, et al. Minimal changes in the systemic immune response after nephrectomy of localized renal masses. Urol Oncol 2014;32(5): 589–600.

29. Zheng K, Tan JM, Wu WZ, et al. Adjuvant dendritic cells vaccine combined with cytokine-induced killer cell therapy after renal cell carcinoma surgery. J BUON 2015;20(2):505–13.

30. Zhan HL, Gao X, Pu XY, et al. A randomized controlled trial of postoperative tumor lysate-pulsed dendritic cells and cytokine-induced killer cells immunotherapy in patients with localized and locally advanced renal cell carcinoma. Chin Med J (Engl) 2012;125(21):3771–7.

31. Galligioni E, Quaia M, Merlo A, et al. Adjuvant immunotherapy treatment of renal carcinoma patients with autologous tumor cells and bacillus Calmette-Guérin: five-year results of a prospective randomized study. Cancer 1996;77:2560–6.

32. Clark JI, Atkins MB, Urba WJ, et al. Adjuvant high-dose bolus interleukin-2 for patients with high-risk renal cell carcinoma: a cytokine working group randomized trial. J Clin Oncol 2003;21:3133–40.

33. Passalacqua R, Caminiti C, Buti S, et al, POLAR-01 Trial Investigators. Adjuvant low-dose interleukin-2 (Il -2) plus interferon-α (IFN-α) in operable renal cell carcinoma (RCC): a phase III, randomized, multicenter trial of the Italian Oncology Group for Clinical Research (GOIRC). J Immunother 2014; 37(9):440–7.

34. Kwak C, Park YH, Jeong CW, et al. No role of adjuvant systemic therapy after complete metastasectomy in metastatic renal cell carcinoma? Urol Oncol 2007;25(4):310–6.

35. Hammers HJ, Plimack ER, Infante JR, et al. Phase I study of nivolumab in combination with ipilimumab in metastatic renal cell carcinoma (mRCC). Ann Oncol 2014;25(Suppl 4):iv361–2.

36. Amin A, Plimack ER, Infante JR, et al. Nivolumab (anti-PD-1; BMS-936558, ONO-4538) in combination with sunitinib or pazopanib in patients (pts) with metastatic renal cell carcinoma (mRCC). J Clin Oncol 2014;32(Suppl) [abstr: 5010].

37. Oudard S, Rixe O, Beuselinck B, et al. A phase II study of the cancer vaccine TG4010 alone and in combination with cytokines in patients with metastatic renal clear-cell carcinoma: clinical and immunological findings. Cancer Immunol Immunother 2011;60:261–71.

38. Amato RJ, Hawkins RE, Kaufman HL, et al. Vaccination of metastatic renal cancer patients with MVA-5T4: a randomized, double-blind, placebo-controlled phase III study. Clin Cancer Res 2010; 16:5539–47.

39. Figlin RA, Nicolette CA, Amin A, et al. Monitoring T-cell responses in a phase II study of AGS-003, an autologous dendritic cell-based therapy in patients with newly diagnosed advanced stage renal cell carcinoma in combination with sunitinib. J Clin Oncol 2011;29(Suppl) [abstr: 2532].

40. Figlin RA, Amin A, Dudek A, et al. Phase II study combining personalized dendritic cell (DC)-based therapy, AGS-003, with sunitinib in metastatic renal cell carcinoma (mRCC). J Clin Oncol 2012; 30(Suppl 5) [abstr: 348].

41. Amin A, Dudek A, Logan T, et al. Prolonged survival with personalized immunotherapy (AGS-003) in combination with sunitinib in unfavorable risk metastatic RCC (mRCC). J Clin Oncol 2013;31(Suppl 6) [abstr: 357].

42. Huland E, Burger A, Fleischer J, et al. Efficacy and safety of inhaled recombinant interleukin-2 in high-risk renal cell cancer patients compared with systemic interleukin-2: an outcome study. Folia Biol (Praha) 2003;49(5):183–90.

43. Coley WB II. Contribution to the knowledge of sarcoma. Ann Surg 1891;14:199–220.

44. Sorbye SW, Kilvaer TK, Valkov A, et al. Prognostic impact of peritumoral lymphocyte infiltration in soft tissue sarcomas. BMC Clin Pathol 2012;12:5.

45. Sorbye SW, Kilvaer T, Valkov A, et al. High expression of CD20+ lymphocytes in soft tissue sarcomas is a positive prognostic indicator. Oncoimmunology 2012;1(1):75–7.

46. Sorbye SW, Kilvaer TK, Valkov A, et al. Prognostic impact of CD57, CD68, M-CSF, CSF-1R, Ki67 and TGF-beta in soft tissue sarcomas. BMC Clin Pathol 2012;12:7.

47. D'Angelo SP, Shoushtari AN, Agaram NP, et al. Prevalence of tumor-infiltrating lymphocytes and PD-L1 expression in the soft tissue sarcoma microenvironment. Hum Pathol 2015;46(3):357–65.

48. D'Angelo SP, Tap WD, Schwartz GK, et al. Sarcoma immunotherapy: past approaches and future directions. Sarcoma 2014;2014:391967.

49. Whelan J, Patterson D, Perisoglou M, et al. The role of interferons in the treatment of osteosarcoma. Pediatr Blood Cancer 2010;54(3):350–4.

50. Strander H, Bauer HC, Brosjö O, et al. Long-term adjuvant interferon treatment of human osteosarcoma. A pilot study. Acta Oncol 1995; 34(6):877–80.

51. Müller CR, Smeland S, Bauer HC, et al. Interferon-alpha as the only adjuvant treatment in high-grade osteosarcoma: long term results of the Karolinska Hospital series. Acta Oncol 2005;44(5):475–80.

52. Winkler K, Beron G, Kotz R, et al. Neoadjuvant chemotherapy for osteogenic sarcoma: results of a cooperative German/Austrian study. J Clin Oncol 1984;2(6):617–24.

53. Bielack SS, Whelan J, Marina N. MAP plus maintenance pegylated interferon α-2b (MAPIfn) versus MAP alone in patients with resectable high-grade osteosarcoma and good histologic response to preoperative MAP: first results of the EURAMOS-1 "good response" randomization. J Clin Oncol 2013;31(Supplement) [abstract: LBA10504].

54. Meyers PA, Schwartz CL, Krailo MD, et al, Children's Oncology Group. Osteosarcoma: the addition of muramyl tripeptide to chemotherapy improves overall survival–a report from the Children's Oncology Group. J Clin Oncol 2008;26(4):633–8.

55. Chou AJ, Kleinerman ES, Krailo MD, et al, Children's Oncology Group. Addition of muramyl tripeptide to chemotherapy for patients with newly diagnosed metastatic osteosarcoma: a report from the Children's Oncology Group. Cancer 2009;115(22):5339–48.

56. Anderson PM, Meyers P, Kleinerman E, et al. Mifamurtide in metastatic and recurrent osteosarcoma: a patient access study with pharmacokinetic, pharmacodynamic, and safety assessments. Pediatr Blood Cancer 2014;61(2):238–44.

57. Goldberg JM, Fisher DE, Demetri GD, et al. Biologic activity of autologous, granulocyte-macrophage colony-stimulating factor secreting alveolar soft-part sarcoma and clear cell sarcoma vaccines. Clin Cancer Res 2015;21(14):3178–86.

58. Robbins PF, Morgan RA, Feldman SA, et al. Tumor regression in patients with metastatic synovial cell sarcoma and melanoma using genetically engineered lymphocytes reactive with NY-ESO-1. J Clin Oncol 2011;29(7):917–24.

59. Huang X, Park H, Greene J, et al. IGF1R- and ROR1-specific CAR T cells as a potential therapy for high risk sarcomas. PLoS One 2015;10(7):e0133152.

60. Ahmed N, Brawley VS, Hegde M, et al. Human Epidermal growth factor receptor 2 (HER2)-specific chimeric antigen receptor-modified T cells for the immunotherapy of HER2-positive sarcoma. J Clin Oncol 2015;33(15):1688–96.

61. Galon J, Costes A, Sanchez-Cabo F, et al. Type, density, and location of immune cells within human colorectal tumors predict clinical outcome. Science 2006;313:1960–4.

62. Vermorken JB, Claessen AM, van Tinteren H, et al. Active specific immunotherapy for stage II and stage III human colon cancer: a randomized trial. Lancet 1999;353:345–50.

63. Ockert D, Schirrmacher V, Beck N, et al. Newcastle disease virus-infected intact autologous tumor cell vaccine for adjuvant active specific immunotherapy of resected colorectal carcinoma. Clin Cancer Res 1996;2:21–8.

64. Schlag P, Manasterski M, Gerneth T, et al. Active specific immunotherapy with Newcastle-disease-virus-modified autologous tumor cells following resection of liver metastases in colorectal cancer, first evaluation of clinical response of a phase II-trial. Cancer Immunol Immunother 1992;35:325–30.

65. Schulze T, Kemmner W, Weitz J, et al. Efficiency of adjuvant active specific immunization with Newcastle disease virus modified tumor cells in colorectal cancer patients following resection of liver metastases: results of a prospective randomized trial. Cancer Immunol Immunother 2009;58:61–9.

66. Posner MC, Niedzwiecki D, Venook AP, et al. A phase II prospective multi-institutional trial of adjuvant active specific immunotherapy following curative resection of colorectal cancer hepatic metastases: cancer and leukemia group B study 89903. Ann Surg Oncol 2008;15:58–64.

67. Barth RJ Jr, Fisher DA, Wallace PK, et al. A randomized trial of ex vivo CD40L activation of a dendritic cell vaccine in colorectal cancer patients: tumor-specific immune responses are associated with improved survival. Clin Cancer Res 2010;16:5548–56.

68. Morse M, Nair S, Mosca P, et al. Immunotherapy with autologous, human dendritic cells transfected with carcinoembryonic antigen mRNA. Cancer Invest 2003;21:341–9.

69. Morse MA, Niedzwiecki D, Marshall JL, et al. A randomized phase II study of immunization with dendritic cells modified with poxvectors encoding CEA and MUC1 compared with the same poxvectors plus GM-CSF for resected metastatic colorectal cancer. Ann Surg 2013;258(6):879–86.

70. Morse MA, Nair S, Fernandez-Casal M, et al. Preoperative mobilization of circulating dendritic cells by Flt3 ligand administration to patients with metastatic colon cancer. J Clin Oncol 2000;18(23):3883–93.

71. Lynch DH. Induction of dendritic cells (DC) by Flt3 ligand (FL) promotes the generation of tumor-specific immune responses in vivo. Crit Rev Immunol 1998;18:99–107.

72. Dolcetti R, Viel A, Doglioni C, et al. High prevalence of activated intraepithelial cytotoxic T lymphocytes and increased neoplastic cell apoptosis in colorectal carcinomas with microsatellite instability. Am J Pathol 1999;154:1805–13.

73. Le DT, Uram JN, Wang H, et al. PD-1 blockade in tumors with mismatch repair deficiency. J Clin Oncol 2015;33(Suppl) [abstr: LBA100].

74. Vansteenkiste JF, Cho B, Vanakesa T, et al. MAGRIT, a double-blind, randomized, placebo-controlled phase III study to assess the efficacy of the recMAGE-A3 + AS15 cancer immunotherapeutic as adjuvant therapy in patients with resected MAGE-A3-positive non-small cell lung cancer (NSCLC). ESMO; 2014 [abstract: 11730]. Availabe at: https://content.webges.com/library/esmo/browse/itinerary/478/2014-09-28#9f9n02uR.

75. Langer CJ. Emerging immunotherapies in the treatment of non-small cell lung cancer (NSCLC): the role of immune checkpoint inhibitors. Am J Clin Oncol 2015;38(4):422–30.

76. Mittendorf EA, Clifton GT, Holmes JP, et al. Final report of the phase I/II clinical trial of the E75 (nelipepimut-S) vaccine with booster inoculations to prevent disease recurrence in high-risk breast cancer patients. Ann Oncol 2014;25(9):1735–42.

77. Wang Y, Yang M, Yu Q, et al. Recombinant bacillus Calmette-Guérin in urothelial bladder cancer immunotherapy: current strategies. Expert Rev Anticancer Ther 2015;15(1):85–93.

78. Powles T, Eder JP, Fine GD, et al. MPDL3280A (anti-PD-L1) treatment leads to clinical activity in metastatic bladder cancer. Nature 2014;515(7528):558–62.

Is Surgery Warranted for Oligometastatic Disease?

Tom Treasure, MD, MS, FRCS, FRCP[a],*, Fergus Macbeth, MA, DM, FRCR, FRCP[b]

KEYWORDS

- Lung metastasectomy • Colorectal cancer • Clinical effectiveness • Citation network analysis
- Ablation

KEY POINTS

- The removal or ablation of pulmonary metastases for carcinoma (especially colorectal) is being increasingly carried out with the aim of improving survival.
- Lung metastases from carcinoma are rarely the primary cause of death.
- Observational studies cannot reliably show the long term effectiveness of pulmonary metastasectomy; there have been no randomised trials.
- There have been randomised trials of monitoring strategies to detect and treat metastatic disease earlier: they have shown no survival benefit.
- Pulmonary metastasectomy with curative intent is not justifiable on the currently available evidence.

It is now widely believed that the resection of metastases from the lung of a patient with cancer is a useful procedure and one that improves survival. That there is an issue of *Thoracic Surgery Clinics* devoted to the topic is a testament to this belief. The new less-invasive techniques of ablating metastases and the increased use of videothoracoscopy seem to be making this approach even more popular. This article strongly challenges the belief in clinical effectiveness and demonstrates that metastasectomy is supported neither by a sound biological rationale nor by any good evidence. Reasons are suggested why this unfounded belief has become so prevalent.

The authors are not dogmatic nihilists. The noted British economist John Maynard Keynes once wrote, "When my information changes, I alter my conclusions. What do you do, sir?" The authors' current position is based on a careful consideration of the current evidence and if this evidence changes the authors are prepared to change their minds.

Colorectal cancer is currently the most common histology for lung metastasectomy. For most of this article, unless otherwise stated, colorectal cancer is used to make generalizable points that apply to the management of other carcinomas that have similar overall behavior. Sarcoma and germ cell tumors may be different[1] and are discussed in Chapter 7 by Duykhanh Ceppa. Metastases are rarely symptomatic and usually remains so even in later stages of colorectal cancer. Policies of surveillance are specifically designed to detect asymptomatic metastatic disease. Furthermore, the practice of metastasectomy is selective and the rare metastases that cause symptoms generally fall outside the criteria for lung metastasectomy performed with intent to cure.

THE PARADIGM OF CANCER SURGERY WITH INTENT TO CURE

The paradigm of curative cancer surgery used to be simple. The cancer had to be localized so that the surgeon could perform an operation that successfully removed it with clear margins, confirming by microscopy that the intent to leave no residual primary disease was achieved. Local lymph nodes could be included in what was intended to be an en bloc

a Clinical Operational Research Unit, 4 Taviton Street, University College London, London WC1H 0BT, United Kingdom; b Wales Cancer Trials Unit, 6th Floor, Neuadd Meirionnydd, University Hospital of Wales, Heath Park, Cardiff CF14 4YS, United Kingdom
* Corresponding author.
E-mail address: tom.treasure@gmail.com

Thorac Surg Clin 26 (2016) 79–90
http://dx.doi.org/10.1016/j.thorsurg.2015.09.010
1547-4127/16/$ – see front matter © 2016 Elsevier Inc. All rights reserved.

curative resection. This might also include regional nodes taken with the intervening tissue in continuity, but the presence of more remote lymph nodes and blood-borne metastases (M1 disease) was believed to make surgery futile or unavailing. Of the two, the authors prefer to use the word unavailing which retains a sense of a well-intentioned operation even if surgeons' efforts may have not been effective.

The Halsted operation for breast cancer followed this paradigm of taking the whole breast, with the primary cancer within it, and the draining lymph nodes, in continuity. The operation held sway for 80 years and any less radical surgery was regarded as undertreatment, which compromised the chance of cure. The Halsted paradigm was en bloc clearance of all disease and extending the operation to remove as many lymph nodes as possible gave the best chance of cure. Radical mastectomy was challenged by Bernard Fisher in 1970 in a 50-page treatise.[2]

The abbreviated version of the history[3] is that radical mastectomy was definitively overturned by the results of a randomized trial published in 1981 the New England Journal of Medicine.[4] Even prior to that study, however, many surgeons had already desisted from performing radical mastectomy. When invited to write a state-of-the-art article published in 1978 in the British Medical Journal, Harold Ellis, a highly regarded surgical teacher, never mentioned radical mastectomy.[5] Radical mastectomy was already on the wane. This illustrates a corollary that unless and until there is sufficient uncertainty to allow a balance of opposing views, now known as group equipoise, controlled trials with treatment assignment by randomization are not ethically possible.

The implication of all this is that breast cancer (and probably many other common cancers) may well be a systemic condition earlier than was previously considered and that extensive, often mutilating, surgery does not achieve the hoped-for cure and is not in patients' interests. So it is unlikely that removing a few radiologically visible metastases from the lung changes the course of the disease. Removing as many as 124 metastases from the lungs, as has been reported, seems to the authors to be beyond reason.[6]

The paradigm of resection of the primary and locoregional disease en bloc now seems to be abandoned and replaced by a sincerely held belief that resecting a few liver or lung metastases can result in durable disease-free survival. From basic principles, it seems implausible that survival can be substantially altered by piecemeal removal of blood-borne metastases from a destination organ such as the lung. It is not clear to the authors that there is any substantial evidence to justify this change. Doubts about effectiveness of lung metastasectomy were published in a well-reasoned but rarely cited article 35 years ago.[7,8]

DEFINING TERMS: OLIGOMETASTASIS

Oligometastatic disease is now a popular term but what exactly does it mean? As argued in this article, it means nothing more than what the word itself says: few metastases. The authors conclude that the oligometastatic state is a therapeutic opportunity where there are few enough metastases to consider ablating or removing them all in turn. There is nothing wrong in itself with defining a disease by the treatment available. There is an excellent precedent in the case of end-stage renal disease (ESRD), which is a diagnostic label, or perhaps better, a frame,[9] for a disease that, once diagnosed, attracts federal funding for renal replacement therapy (Box 1).[10]

The term oligometastasis seems to have appeared for the first time in the literature in 1995.[11] The article's authors, Hellman and Weichselbaum, introduce their exposition of the metastatic state with reference to Halsted and breast cancer. The Halsted theory, according to their account, proposed that cancer spread is orderly, extending in a contiguous fashion from the primary tumor through the lymphatics to the lymph nodes and then to distant sites.[11] The investigators use the words, "theory" and "hypothesis", in their introduction before proposing the existence of a clinical significant state of oligometastases.

Box 1
Framing disease

History of renal failure from dropsy to ESRD[13]

- From ancient times to the eighteenth century, dropsy was a clinical diagnosis for a body overloaded with water.

- From the 1820s, Richard Bright of Guy's Hospital in London recognized that some patients with dropsy had albumen in their urine and shriveled kidneys, which distinguished them from those with heart disease as the cause of what is now called edema, and this was known as Bright disease.

- People who have kidney disease necessitating renal replacement therapy now receive the diagnosis of ESRD, which since 1972 entitles them to centrally funded renal replacement therapy.[10]

Data from Rosenberg CE, Golden J. Framing disease: studies in cultural history. New Brunswick (NJ): Rutgers University Press; 1992.

Considering how commonly the words, *oligo-metastasis* and *oligometastases*, are used in the argot of tumor boards and multidisciplinary team meetings, the number of articles addressing the subject are few (**Fig. 1**). The term is used increasingly in the literature but largely as a flag of convenience. Particularly in prostate cancer, a convention has been adopted that the cutoff for the oligometastatic state is 5 or fewer metastases. The authors are unaware of a biological rationale for this. It is an example of a diagnostic frame defined by the practical considerations of how the disease is to be treated. In the intervening twenty years since the introduction of the concept of the oligometastatic state, increased spacial resolution of existing imaging, and the introduction of new methods, has resulted in the ability to detect more of the metastases that are present. Alongside increasing the ability to detect previously unexpected metastases, more crucially, PET has added greater power to demonstrate the absence of metastases, at least those above a critical size-times-activity threshold, with the ability to limit with more confidence the likelihood of there being many more occult metastases when embarking on treating the few. Thus, oligometastasis is defined by the absence of more than can be dealt with by ablations and/or resection.

As with any new investigation that increases sensitivity of detection, PET has caused stage shift. Previously occult metastases are detected and a tranche of patients are excluded by staging drift. Patients deemed oligometastatic by PET will have a better prognosis than similar patients would have had in the pre-PET era. If staging drift coincides with introduction of ablative therapies, better survival than in previous reports may be attributed to the therapy rather than to a more favorable treated patient group defined by PET.

If metastases could be seen down to a very few cells and monitored continuously, then it could be argued that there must always have been a first and second metastasis, but such theorising does not help in the practical management of patients. The number is arbitrary and based on what might reasonably be attempted by ablative therapies. It is not based on anything to do with their biology but on the belief that there are few enough of them to ablate.[12]

The term oligometastasis may be a useful diagnostic frame[11] with 5 or fewer metastases as an operational definition as to what might be treatable by ablative therapies, thus providing a therapeutic opportunity.[13] But is this really true? Five or fewer may be a useful cutoff for feasibility of treatments with radiofrequency ablation or stereotactic body radiotherapy (SBRT), but does this apply to surgery for lung metastases? A patient with 5 metastases might have all 5 in 1 lobe, making lobectomy a pragmatic approach. On the other hand, there may be 1 in each lobe and all 5 lobes cannot be removed. Their removal may be possible by videothoracoscopy but it becomes clear that the treatment on offer is then being driven by practicalities and technical craft, not science.[14–16] As many as 124 lung metastases have been removed from a patient with breast cancer.[6] The investigators include this as a case of complete resection, but it is absurd to believe that there is not a 125th lurking somewhere beyond the resolution of current imaging.

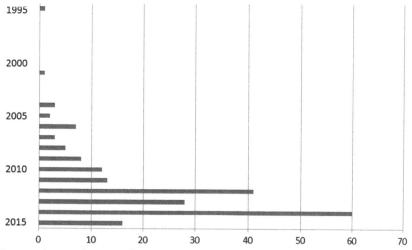

Fig. 1. Over 20 years, the search term <oligometas*> appeared 200 times in the titles of articles and peaked at 60 in 2014. The count had reached 55 for 2015 by October.

If there were a biologically determined oligometastatic state, this might be revealed by discontinuity in the distribution curve resulting in a multimodal distribution. It seems more likely from everyday observation that the distribution of metastatic number is continuous and would have a Poisson distribution. Most tumors that metastasize tend to produce numerous metastases limited in their eventual number by their cumulative mass, resulting in the death of the patient. There is a tail in the Poisson distribution, tapering out to the few patients with just 3, 2, or a solitary metastasis.

It is has been suggested, based on work with microRNAs, that oligometastasis and polymetastasis are distinct entities at the clinical and molecular levels.[17] So far the authors are unconvinced that this is a clinically useful analysis but await further evidence.

DEFINING TERMS: WARRANTED

British English speakers are concerned with making themselves clear in international English and need to define the words given in a title.[18] *Warranted* means that a treatment is justified and that there is reasonable expectation that it provides the desired health gain for the patient.

DEFINING TERMS: EFFICACY AND EFFECTIVENESS

To be warranted for an individual, treatments should be effective, that is, they achieve the desired clinical outcome and resulting health gain. The words *efficacy* and *effectiveness* are not readily distinguished in everyday English and are often used interchangeably. Any subtle differences in their meanings in everyday speech are lost in usage determined by context and culture. It is worth understanding, however, how these words convey different meanings in the language of evidence-based medicine (EBM)[19] (**Fig. 2**).

The efficacy of a clinical procedure means that a subsequent pathologic or biological change can be observed. Effectiveness implies that there is a useful and relevant clinical outcome resulting from the intervention. That the target metastasis is removed with microscopically clear margins (R0) is evidence of efficacy. Ablative techniques, such as radiofrequency ablation and stereotactic ablative radiotherapy, which have the theoretic advantage of being less invasive and harmful, do not pass the test of efficacy against the standards set by surgery. The destruction of tissue extending beyond the margin of the cancer cannot be determined.[20]

So what then is the effectiveness of procedures aimed at removing or ablating metastases?

PALLIATIVE SURGERY

The authors believe that treating or removing specific metastases to relieve or prevent symptoms is appropriate provided that each case is taken on its merits and the balance of benefit and harm considered. But lung metastases are rarely symptomatic unless so widespread as to compromise lung function and by definition not oligometastatic.

SURGERY INTENDED TO CURE

A policy of advocating metastasectomy is based on the presumption that the removal of the metastasis has survival benefit. In an ideal case, the metastasis is the only residual disease or other sites of disease are within the overall plan for curative treatment. Surgical removal of the lung metastases is curative in that sense. That is, why one of the standard criteria has been from the earliest days that there should be no cancer elsewhere, one of Thomford's time-honored criteria.[21]

Cure is a small word on a big mission. A sufficient definition of cure might be to live a decent length of time and to die free of a particular

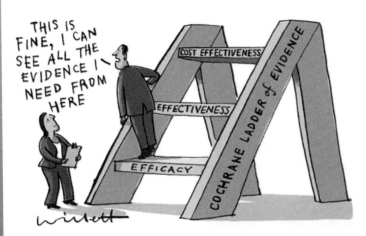

Fig. 2. Efficacy: can it work? Effectiveness: does it work? Cost effectiveness: is it worth it? Evidence steps on the Cochrane staircase. (*From* Jarvinen TL, Sievanen H, Kannus P, et al. The true cost of pharmacologic disease prevention. BMJ 2011;342:d2175; with permission.)

cancer, of some other cause. In follow-up of 1447 patients were recruited into a trial carcinoembryonic antigen (CEA) monitoring from 1982 to 1993. There was a review of death certification in 2013, 20 to 31 years after primary surgery.[22] Many of those patients met the criteria for cure after primary resection. They died many years later with no documented evidence of cancer. There were no survivors among those operated for recurrence. It is admittedly weak evidence from an earlier era, but it is known from contemporary practice that in a majority of cases the disease recurs in the lung or elsewhere and commonly both.[23–27] Patients go on to die of the disease. Although surgery may be undertaken under the notional heading of curative intent, this fails much more often that it succeeds.

SURGERY TO IMPROVE SURVIVAL

Is lung metastasectomy effective in improving survival – making patients live longer even if not cured? When a mechanistically plausible intervention self-evidently, promptly, and consistently alters the course of events, observational evidence has customarily been relied on.[28,29] Surgeons know examples: relieving tension pneumothorax, controlling exsanguinating hemorrhage, and removing a cataract.

Metastasectomy meets none of these criteria. Because patients rarely die as a direct result of lung metastases, the self-evident cause-and-effect relationship is not there. Lung metastases are rarely if ever removed to avert impending death. Candidates for metastasectomy have generally been expected to live with the metastases for some period of time, so the time relationship between metastasectomy and still being alive (that is, not having died yet) is lost. Survival results are routinely presented as 5-year survival rates or median survival, ideally with a range (typically interquartile) to indicate the distribution. In isolation these are of limited value. Most patients go on to die of the cancer and many have lung recurrence. In the absence of controls, it cannot be known whether their survival is longer or shorter than it otherwise would have been.

These patients also have other therapies, including effective chemotherapy. It is also is known well that there is wide variation in natural survival with cancer. Amid all this noise, the signal created by the metastasectomy cannot be reliably discerned.[28] In the absence of a control group or other robust comparator, all that clinicians rely on is the clinical judgment as to how long this patient would have lived without the metastasectomy. That is not the same as knowing how long

an average patient might have lived with cancer of the same extent. There is a readiness on the part of surgeons to attribute all 5-year survival to an effect of metastasectomy as if none would have lived otherwise. It is known that there are some 5-year survivors in the tail end of all cancer survival curves[30,31]; so if there is a difference, a higher survival rate in those who have had a lung metastasectomy, only some of the difference might be due to metastasectomy. The surgeon cannot claim all of it as a treatment effect.

A QUESTION OF ATTRIBUTION: EFFECT OF SURGERY OR OF SELECTION FOR SURGERY?

In successive multivariate analyses of lung metastasectomy for colorectal cancer, fewer metastases and longer intervals between the primary cancer operation and lung metastasectomy have been associated with higher 5-year survival rates.[23,25–27] In colorectal cancer, a further favorable factor is nonelevation of CEA. These are general prognostic factors in colorectal cancer. The distinction between prognostic and predictive factors is an important one.[32] Prognostic features apply irrespective of treatment. Patients with these favorable prognostic features are in the long surviving tail of the survival distribution curves irrespective of what treatment is given. Predictive factors are those that indicate which of patients in a group are likely to respond to a particular treatment, such as receptor status in breast cancer.

In the Thames Cancer Registry for patients with stage 4 colorectal cancer at diagnosis, there were more than 5% of patients still alive at 5 years in an analysis performed in 2007.[31] A simple mathematical model developed as part of the European Society of Thoracic Surgeons Lung Metastasectomy Project shows that it is possible based on 2 factors to select a group of 25 of 300 patients, including 10 of the 15 natural survivors (**Fig. 3**). This replicates the 40% 5-year survival reported in the most series. The degree of selection (25/300, or approximately 8%) is overgenerous. Fewer than 3% were selected in a large prospective registry study, capturing approximately 60% of colorectal lung metastasectomy patients in a 2-year period in Spain.[33] Survival attributed to lung metastasectomy might be no more than a mirage.[34]

Recognition of this evidence is important because it is known that survival is poor if the selection factors identified over many years are not adhered to. The conclusion from the joint Memorial Sloan Kettering Cancer Center and Duke University series of 378 patients was, "Medical management alone should be considered standard for patients who have both three or more pulmonary metastases

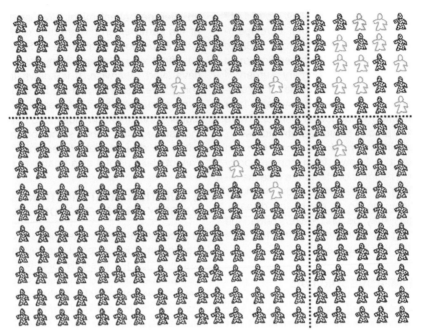

Fig. 3. A pictorial representation of a selection process; 300 patients are ordered by 2 criteria, which, in addition to being criteria for selection, are prognostic factors for survival regardless of intervention. For all patients, there are 15/300 5-year survivors (5%). In this illustration, selecting these 2 criteria (*dotted lines*) gives a group with of 25 patients, including 10 survivors, a rate of 40% survival (patients depicted in smaller square in the top right hand corner). Cancer teams are able to select the more likely survivors and if they are selected for surgery a group is created with an inevitably higher survival rate that might erroneously be attributed to surgery whereas it is a feature of selection. (*From* Utley M, Treasure T. Interpreting data from surgical follow-up studies: the role of modeling. J Thorac Oncol 2010;5:S201; with permission.)

and less than 1 year DFI," because there were no survivors outside these limits.[24] Even more stringent selection should be applied according to a recent meta-analysis of 2925 patients.[27] Patients with more than 1 metastasis, an interval of less than 3 years, and any elevation of CEA had a doubled hazard ratio for each of the criteria breached.

COLORECTAL CANCER AND THE DRIVE TOWARD METASTASECTOMY

With respect to colorectal cancer there was an explicit drive to solve the problem of recurrent abdominal and liver recurrence (**Fig. 4**). The concept behind the policy of second-look surgery, promulgated from the 1950s by Wangensteen and colleagues,[35] in Minneapolis, Minnesota, was that any residual but invisible cancer would grow and at a second operation after an interval it could be seen and palpated and possibly excised, providing a second chance of cure. This was applied in all patients in whom positive lymph nodes had been found at the primary resection.

Approximately 6 months later, while the patients were asymptomatic and without any clinically evident disease, they were operated on again and

any cancer found was removed. If cancer had been found, the patients were scheduled for 2 or more further looks, up to 6 further abdominal operations, "before the abdomen was free of cancer." This second-look policy produced some cures but entailed such high rates of unproductive laparotomy and disturbing operative mortality that it did not gain acceptance. Despite these results, the strategy is still used.[36]

A more precise method of locating patients was the CEA assay. This led to the CEA Second-Look (CEASL) trial, with joint trans-Atlantic Funding from National Institutes of Health in the United States and the Cancer Research Campaign in the United Kingdom.[22] The trial recruited from 1982 to 1993. The protocol at second-look laparotomy included full mobilization of the liver.

While CEASL was recruiting, reports of survival after liver resection began to appear from the Mayo Clinic[37,38] and from the Registry of Hepatic Metastases.[39,40] The idea of a randomized trial was mooted by the Mayo Clinic group, including a power calculation.[41] The possible effect size in terms of 5-year survival (30% vs near 0%) would have required as few as 36 patients. The idea was trumped by institutional observational data

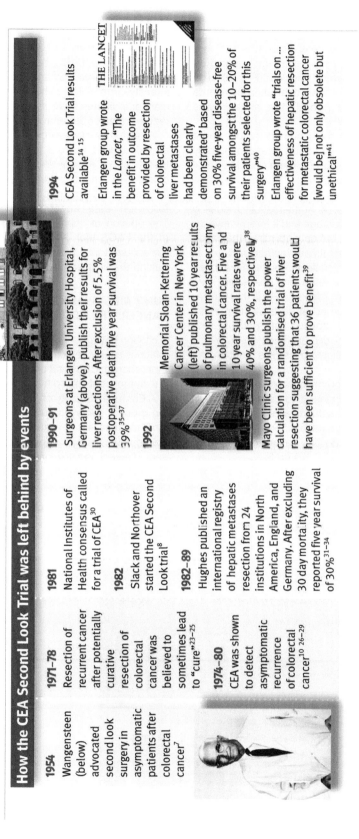

Fig. 4. Footsteps on the route to hepatic resection for metastatic colorectal cancer. (*From* Treasure T, Monson K, Fiorentino F, et al. Operating to remove recurrent colorectal cancer: have we got it right? BMJ 2014;348:18–20; with permission.)

from the University Hospital in Erlangen, Germany.[42,43] The CEASL trial had found no increase in survival from CEA-triggered second-look surgery but an excess of deaths,[44,45] but the manuscript was never sent for publication and the CEA data were shelved (**Fig. 5**). The research question had been overtaken by events and the impetus to publish the answer was lost.[46]

It was at this time the landmark article about 10-year results from pulmonary metastasectomy for colorectal cancer was published from Memorial Sloan Kettering Cancer Center.[47] The previous discussion about the effect of selection applies in review of those results. A mathematical modeling study using the cancer stage and interoperative interval data from those 144 patients raises the possibility that survival without lung metastasectomy in such highly selected patients might have been much better than assumed and the effect size commensurately lower. The key point is that the patients were early stage at the time of the primary resection and the comparison with patients who were stage 4 at the time of registration was invalid.[48] Many subsequent follow-up studies contain the same flaw.

The literature on lung metastasectomy for colorectal cancer has continued to grow.[8] A citation network analysis shows that there is repeated citation of those who share each other's views. Those who take a different view are conveniently ignored and left off the citation list[49] (**Fig. 6**).

The research question of the recently published Follow-up After Colorectal Surgery (FACS) trial was whether intensive surveillance with CEA, CT, or both resulted in a survival advantage compared with neither and only clinical follow-up.[50] Intensive surveillance led to an earlier diagnosis of recurrence, as did CEASL, but there was no survival advantage. There was an excess of deaths in the intensive arm which, although not reaching significance, indicates there might be a detrimental effect from major but unavailing surgery.

When lung metastasectomy was among the recommendations in from the National Institute for Health and Care Excellence guideline, the only citation was an article from the University Hospital in Erlangen, Germany dealing with observational follow-up data about liver metastasectomy.[51] The opinion of John Primrose, chief investigator of the FACS trial, was, "the state of the art on metastasectomy in thoracic surgery is a decade behind that in liver surgery."[52]

LUNG METASTASECTOMY FOR COLORECTAL CANCER: THE STATE OF THE EVIDENCE

A citation network analysis shows the way in which citations are repeated of those whose views the authors share and noncitation of those who disagree.[49] The authors call this "a frenzy of mutual citation."[8]

A European Society of Thoracic Surgeons working group[53] surveyed surgeons for their views on lung metastasectomy and found that many surgeons saw no limit to how many metastases they should resect and how often they should reoperate. Surveys are not reliable measures of actual practice or outcomes but a survey is the best and only way of

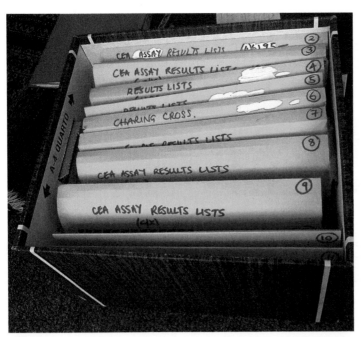

Fig. 5. The files of CEA results in 1447 patients, abandoned in a cupboard for 15 years.

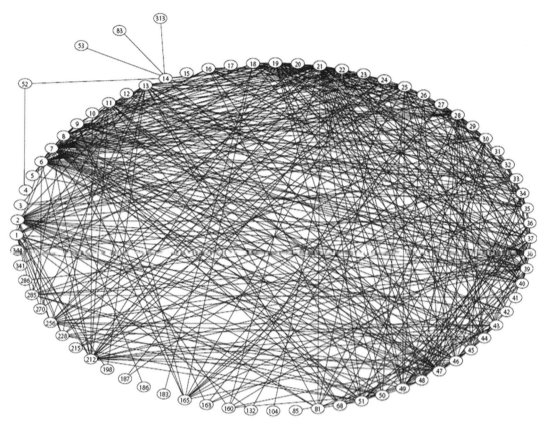

Fig. 6. A citation network of lung metastasectomy for colorectal cancer. (*From* Fiorentino F, Vasilakis C, Treasure T. Clinical reports of pulmonary metastasectomy for colorectal cancer: a citation network analysis. Br J Cancer 2011;104:1087; with permission.)

discovering attitudes and beliefs. In the absence of evidence there is wide variance. The leaders of the European Society of Thoracic Surgeons working group concluded, "Evidence fell well short of Evidence Based Medicine standards and robust guidance could not be produced on this basis."

LUNG METASTASECTOMY FOR SARCOMA: THE STATE OF THE EVIDENCE

From the perspective of EBM, there is also lack of secure evidence for metastasectomy for sarcoma. Because it may only metastasize to lung and it tends to affect the young, a particular view has been taken about it. A systematic review revealed, however, the shortcomings in clarity of objectives and lack of control data (discussed previously).[30] There is, however, the possibility of uncertainty among those thoracic surgeons who are referred these patients.[54] The authors view the following as an important and timely statement:

Future randomized prospective studies are warranted, particularly in patients with a poor risk profile, to define whether any

benefit is derived from lung metastasectomy compared with other local therapies or no resection. In the absence of control (nonoperative) data, quantifying the difference in survival among patients who have undergone metastasectomy and attributing it to surgical resection may not be accurate because there is a selection bias for lung metastasectomy.[55]

WHERE IS LUNG METASTASECTOMY HEADING?

Surgical removal of lung metastases may be a 3-way negotiation between oncologist, patient, and thoracic surgeon. The ensuing scenario is familiar. It is assumed that patients place a high value on life at any cost but they may not have been prepared for the adverse heath consequences or the burden of what may turn out to be a bankrupting sequence of investigations, treatments and interventions.[56,57]

Belief in lung metastasectomy is put forward as unassailable. For example:

Survival of patients with metastatic CRC (mCRC) has improved in the past decade, mainly as a result of more-effective chemotherapy regimens. Obviously, surgical resection of the primary tumor and all metastatic disease also improves survival.[58]

There are good reasons for managing the primary cancer to spare the patient obstruction, perforation, bleeding, tenesmus, fistula, and pain. Those are desirable goals, based on observational data and clinical experience, even if survival is not extended. But where does "obviously" come from? It seems to obviate considering evidence. That "all" metastases can be detected, located, and resected is intrinsically unlikely and needs to be proved clinically effective as a strategy. The entreaty to use words that count and numbers that speak does not seem an unreasonable starting point.[59]

Perhaps even more worrying is this assertion:

The surgical management of colorectal liver metastases (CRLMs) was a paradigm change in the management of metastatic disease and is one of the greatest advances in surgical practice of recent times.[60]

The statement was repeated in a further article that takes the argument to the third step of the Cochrane staircase (see **Fig. 2**) and unjustifiably claims cost utility without any reliable comparative data:

The development of surgical resection as a widely adopted treatment for CRLMs was a paradigm change in the management of metastatic disease, and is one of the most exciting advances in surgical practice in recent times.[61]

When strategies for early detection with a view to resection of metastatic disease have been put to the test in randomized controlled trials, they have shown no benefit and an excess of harm.[22,50] The authors' contribution to resolving this problem is to run the Pulmonary Metastasectomy in Colorectal Cancer trial. It is as far as the authors know the first and only existing trial to test effectiveness of lung metastasectomy.

WHY IS THERE IS ENTHUSIASM FOR METASTASECTOMY?

In the era of EBM, there is a unwarranted level of belief in a procedure for which there is weak evidence. The authors believe that it results from an understandable inclination to do the best for patients. The development of metastases after so-called curative treatment can be seen as a failure. The improvement in imaging technology with better CT scans and PET has also meant that small-volume metastases can be detected at a time when a patient is still asymptomatic and fit enough for potentially toxic interventions. If metastases are looked for and then found, the reasonable expectation is that something can and should be done about them. Pandora's box is open.

A common justification for the removal of metastases is that the knowledge that they are there may cause psychological distress, a real symptom that may be relieved by their removal. Although it is a commonly used justification for metastasectomy, the authors are unaware of any studies confirming or quantifying the health gain. There have been no psychiatrists or psychologists among the investigators of the many articles on surgery of metastases thus far reviewed.[8,25,30,62]

There is also the natural temperament of surgeons – their desire to do something. As John Wennberg has written in relation to the observed variation in the rates of tonsillectomy: "Few surgeons are hesitant believers in the efficacy of the operations they perform, nor do they doubt their clinical necessity."[63] But perhaps all those involved in advising patients about whether or not they should undergo pulmonary metastasectomy should remember the words of Iain Chalmers, founder of the Cochrane Collaboration: "A prerequisite for constructive debate about uncertainties about the effects of treatment is a greater willingness among professionals and the public to admit and discuss them, combined with the humility to acknowledge that good intentions alone have not protected patients from the unintended harmful effects of treatments."[64]

REFERENCES

1. Treasure T, Milosevic M, Fiorentino F, et al. Pulmonary metastasectomy: what is the practice and where is the evidence for effectiveness? Thorax 2014;69:946–9.
2. Fisher B. The surgical dilemma in the primary therapy of invasive breast cancer: a critical appraisal. Curr Probl Surg 1970;7:2–53.
3. Berwick DM. The science of improvement. JAMA 2008;299:1182–4.
4. Veronesi U, Saccozzi R, Del Vecchio M, et al. Comparing radical mastectomy with quadrantectomy, axillary dissection, and radiotherapy in patients with small cancers of the breast. N Engl J Med 1981;305:6–11.
5. Ellis H. If I had... If my wife had cancer of the breast. Br Med J 1978;1:896–7.
6. Rolle A, Pereszlenyi A, Koch R, et al. Is surgery for multiple lung metastases reasonable? A total of 328 consecutive patients with multiple-laser

metastasectomies with a new 1318-nm Nd:YAG laser. J Thorac Cardiovasc Surg 2006;131:1236–42.

7. Aberg T, Malmberg KA, Nilsson B, et al. The effect of metastasectomy: fact or fiction? Ann Thorac Surg 1980;30:378–84.

8. Fiorentino F, Vasilakis C, Treasure T. Clinical reports of pulmonary metastasectomy for colorectal cancer: a citation network analysis. Br J Cancer 2011;104: 1085–97.

9. Rosenberg CE, Golden J. Framing disease: studies in cultural history. New Brunswick (NJ): Rutgers University Press; 1992.

10. Rettig RA. Special treatment–the story of Medicare's ESRD entitlement. N Engl J Med 2011;364:596–8.

11. Hellman S, Weichselbaum RR. Oligometastases. J Clin Oncol 1995;13:8–10.

12. Treasure T. Oligometastatic cancer: an entity, a useful concept, or a therapeutic opportunity? J R Soc Med 2012;105:242–6.

13. Peitzman Steven J. From bright's disease to end-stage renal failure. In: Rosenberg CE, Golden J, editors. Framing disease. Philadelphia: Rutgers; 1992. p. 3–19.

14. Molnar TF, Gebitekin C, Turna A. What are the considerations in the surgical approach in pulmonary metastasectomy? J Thorac Oncol 2010;5: S140–4.

15. Venuta F, Rolle A, Anile M, et al. Techniques used in lung metastasectomy. J Thorac Oncol 2010;5: S145–50.

16. Migliore M, Jakovic R, Hensens A, et al. Extending surgery for pulmonary metastasectomy: what are the limits? J Thorac Oncol 2010;5:S155–60.

17. Lussier YA, Khodarev NN, Regan K, et al. Oligo- and polymetastatic progression in lung metastasis(es) patients is associated with specific MicroRNAs. PLoS One 2012;7:e50141.

18. Furuse A. International English. Available at: http://www.ctsnet.org/doc/6672.

19. Jarvinen TL, Sievanen H, Kannus P, et al. The true cost of pharmacological disease prevention. BMJ 2011;342:d2175.

20. Palma DA, Salama JK, Lo SS, et al. The oligometastatic state-separating truth from wishful thinking. Nat Rev Clin Oncol 2014;11(9):549–57.

21. Thomford NR, Woolner L, Clagett O. The surgical treatment of metastatic tumours in the lung. J Thorac Cardiovasc Surg 1965;49:357–63.

22. Treasure T, Monson K, Fiorentino F, et al. The CEA Second-Look Trial: a randomised controlled trial of carcinoembryonic antigen prompted reoperation for recurrent colorectal cancer. BMJ Open 2014;4: e004385.

23. Pfannschmidt J, Dienemann H, Hoffmann H. Surgical resection of pulmonary metastases from colorectal cancer: a systematic review of published series. Ann Thorac Surg 2007;84:324–38.

24. Onaitis MW, Petersen RP, Haney JC, et al. Prognostic factors for recurrence after pulmonary resection of colorectal cancer metastases. Ann Thorac Surg 2009;87:1684–8.

25. Fiorentino F, Hunt I, Teoh K, et al. Pulmonary metastasectomy in colorectal cancer: a systematic review and quantitative synthesis. J R Soc Med 2010;103:60–6.

26. Pfannschmidt J, Hoffmann H, Dienemann H. Reported outcome factors for pulmonary resection in metastatic colorectal cancer. J Thorac Oncol 2010; 5:S172–8.

27. Gonzalez M, Poncet A, Combescure C, et al. Risk factors for survival after lung metastasectomy in colorectal cancer patients: a systematic review and meta-analysis. Ann Surg Oncol 2013;20:572–9.

28. Glasziou P, Chalmers I, Rawlins M, et al. When are randomised trials unnecessary? Picking signal from noise. BMJ 2007;334:349–51.

29. Fiorentino F, Treasure T. Pulmonary metastasectomy: are observational studies sufficient evidence for effectiveness? Ann Thorac Surg 2013; 96:1129–31.

30. Treasure T, Fiorentino F, Scarci M, et al. Pulmonary metastasectomy for sarcoma: a systematic review of reported outcomes in the context of Thames cancer registry data. BMJ Open 2012;2:e001736.

31. Utley M, Treasure T, Linklater K, et al. Better out than in? The resection of pulmonary metastases from colorectal tumours. In: Xie X, Lorca F, Marcon E, editors. Operations research for health care engineering: proceedings of the 33rd International Conference on Operational Research Applied to Health Services. Saint-Etienne (France): Publications de l'Universitaire de Saint-Etienne; 2008. p. 493–500.

32. Simms L, Barraclough H, Govindan R. Biostatistics primer: what a clinician ought to know-prognostic and predictive factors. J Thorac Oncol 2013;8: 808–13.

33. Embun R, Fiorentino F, Treasure T, et al. Pulmonary metastasectomy in colorectal cancer: a prospective study of demography and clinical characteristics of 543 patients in the Spanish colorectal metastasectomy registry (GECMP-CCR). BMJ Open 2013;3: e002787.

34. Huang F, Wu G, Yang K. Oligometastasis and oligo-recurrence: more than a mirage. Radiat Oncol 2014; 9:230.

35. Wangensteen O, Lewis F, Arhelger S, et al. An interim report upon the second look procedure for cancer of the stomach, colon, and rectum and for limited intraperitoneal carcinosis. Surg Gynecol Obstet 1954;99:257–67.

36. Sugarbaker PH. Revised guidelines for second-look surgery in patients with colon and rectal cancer. Clin Transl Oncol 2010;12:621–8.

37. Adson MA, Van Heerden JA, Adson MH, et al. Resection of hepatic metastases from colorectal cancer. Arch Surg 1984;119:647–51.

38. Adson MA. Resection of liver metastases–when is it worthwhile? World J Surg 1987;11:511–20.

39. Hughes K. Registry of hepatic metastases: resection of the liver for colorectal carcinoma metastases: a multi-institutional study of indications for resection. Surgery 1988;103:278–88.

40. Hughes KS, Simon R, Songhorabodi S, et al. Resection of the liver for colorectal carcinoma metastases: a multi-institutional study of patterns of recurrence. Surgery 1986;100:278–84.

41. Rosen CB, Nagorney DM, Taswell HF, et al. Perioperative blood transfusion and determinants of survival after liver resection for metastatic colorectal carcinoma. Ann Surg 1992;216:493–504.

42. Scheele J, Stangl R, Altendorf-Hofmann A, et al. Indicators of prognosis after hepatic resection for colorectal secondaries. Surgery 1991;110:13–29.

43. Scheele J, Altendorf-Hofmann A, Stangl R, et al. Pulmonary resection for metastatic colon and upper rectum cancer. Is it useful? Dis Colon Rectum 1990;33:745–52.

44. Northover J, Houghton J. Post operative CEA monitoring and second-look surgery in colorectal cancer: the effect on survival measured using a multicentre randomised trial (Manuscript). 1994.

45. Northover J, Houghton J, Lennon T. CEA to detect recurrence of colon cancer [Letter]. JAMA 1994;272:31.

46. Treasure T, Monson K, Fiorentino F, et al. Operating to remove recurrent colorectal cancer: have we got it right? BMJ 2014;348:g2085.

47. McCormack PM, Burt ME, Bains MS, et al. Lung resection for colorectal metastases. 10-year results. Arch Surg 1992;127:1403–6.

48. Fiorentino F, Treasure T. Pulmonary metastasectomy for colorectal cancer: Making the case for a randomized controlled trial in the zone of uncertainty. J Thorac Cardiovasc Surg 2013;146:748–52.

49. Greenberg SA. How citation distortions create unfounded authority: analysis of a citation network. BMJ 2009;339:b2680.

50. Primrose JN, Perera R, Gray A, et al. Effect of 3 to 5 years of scheduled CEA and CT follow-up to detect recurrence of colorectal cancer: the FACS randomized clinical trial. JAMA 2014;311:263–70.

51. Stangl R, Altendorf-Hofmann A, Charnley RM, et al. Factors influencing the natural history of colorectal liver metastases. Lancet 1994;343:1405–10.

52. Primrose J, Treasure T, Fiorentino F. Lung metastasectomy in colorectal cancer: is this surgery effective in prolonging life? Respirology 2010;15:742–6.

53. Van Raemdonck D, Friedel G. The European Society of Thoracic Surgeons Lung Metastasectomy Project. J Thorac Oncol 2010;5:S127–9.

54. Treasure T, Macbeth F. Doubt about effectiveness of lung metastasectomy for sarcoma. J Thorac Cardiovasc Surg 2015;149:93–4.

55. Lin AY, Kotova S, Yanagawa J, et al. Risk stratification of patients undergoing pulmonary metastasectomy for soft tissue and bone sarcomas. J Thorac Cardiovasc Surg 2015;149:85–92.

56. Russell RCG, Treasure T. Counting the cost of cancer surgery for advanced and metastatic disease. Br J Surg 2012;99:449–50.

57. Bennett A. The cost of hope. London: Random House; 2012.

58. van de Velde CJ. Surgery: Palliative primary tumour resection in mCRC-debate continues. Nat Rev Clin Oncol 2015;12:129–30.

59. Treasure W. Diagnosis and risk management in primary care: words that count, numbers that speak. London: Radcliffe Publishing; 2011.

60. Roberts KJ, White A, Cockbain A, et al. Performance of prognostic scores in predicting long-term outcome following resection of colorectal liver metastases. Br J Surg 2014;101:856–66.

61. Roberts KJ, Sutton AJ, Prasad KR, et al. Cost-utility analysis of operative versus non-operative treatment for colorectal liver metastases. Br J Surg 2015;102:388–98.

62. Grunhagen D, Jones RP, Treasure T, et al. The history of adoption of hepatic resection for metastatic colorectal cancer: 1984-95. Crit Rev Oncol Hematol 2013;86:222–31.

63. Wennberg J. Commentary: a debt of gratitude to J. Alison Glover. Int J Epidemiol 2008;37:26–9.

64. Chalmers I. Well informed uncertainties about the effects of treatments. BMJ 2004;328:475–6.

Thoracoscopic Management of Pulmonary Metastases

Elliot Servais, MD[a], Scott J. Swanson, MD[b],*

KEYWORDS

- VATS metastasectomy • Thoracoscopic surgery • Pulmonary metastasectomy
- Minimally invasive surgery

KEY POINTS

- Thoracoscopic pulmonary metastasectomy can prolong survival in appropriately selected patients with metastatic disease to the lungs.
- The thoracoscopic approach may decrease immunologic insult, postoperative pain, and hospital stay compared with open approaches.
- With advances in preoperative imaging, only extremely small (<2 mm) lesions are at risk for being missed during thoracoscopic metastasectomy and this is of unclear clinical significance.
- Pulmonary metastases recur in the lungs in up to 53% of patients; repeat thoracoscopic pulmonary metastasectomy is a reasonable strategy to address these recurrent lesions.

INTRODUCTION

Pulmonary metastases represent systemic dissemination of cancer and, as such, often portends poor prognosis. In many settings, the presence of metastases triggers a switch in the treatment priority from aggressive, cure-oriented therapy to palliative strategies. However, investigators have long considered the utility of metastasectomy, particularly for patients in whom the lungs represent the only discernible site of distant disease. Reports of pulmonary metastasectomy producing long-term survivors date back to the early 1940s.[1] Nevertheless, for several decades there was a scarcity of data to support resection of pulmonary metastases and clinicians widely questioned the legitimacy of this strategy.[2]

In 1997, Pastorino and colleagues[3] published a review from the International Registry of Lung Metastases identifying 5206 cases of metastasectomy.

Despite being a retrospective analysis, this article set forth the best evidence yet in support of pulmonary metastasectomy as safe and efficacious. Cell of origin, disease-free interval, complete resectability, and number of metastases were found to predict survival following metastasectomy and have thus become the primary oncologic determinants of a patient's candidacy for surgery. Despite these data, the role for metastasectomy remains a hotly debated topic. Whereas few clinicians would object to resecting a solitary colorectal metastasis in the lung of an otherwise healthy young patient, questions of multiple metastases, repeat metastasectomy, and minimally invasive approaches to metastasectomy are met with far less consensus. Several of these controversies are addressed elsewhere in this issue of *Thoracic Surgery Clinics*. Herein we address the question of surgical approach to metastasectomy and specifically relate the benefits and technical aspects of a

[a] Cardiothoracic Surgery, Brigham and Women's Hospital, Harvard Medical School, 75 Francis Street, Boston, MA 02115, USA; [b] Minimally Invasive Thoracic Surgery, Cancer Affairs, Department of Surgery, Dana-Farber Cancer Institute, Brigham and Women's Hospital, Harvard Medical School, 75 Francis Street, Boston, MA 02115, USA
* Corresponding author.
E-mail address: sjswanson@partners.org

Thorac Surg Clin 26 (2016) 91–97
http://dx.doi.org/10.1016/j.thorsurg.2015.09.011

thoracoscopic approach, which has become our standard technique in most cases.

THORACOSCOPIC PULMONARY METASTASECTOMY

Traditional teaching emphasized bimanual palpation of lung tissue during metastasectomy to ensure the complete resection of all metastatic lesions, specifically including those below the threshold of identification on preoperative imaging.[4,5] To this end, unilateral metastases were classically approached via thoracotomy and bilateral metastases via sternotomy, clamshell thoracotomy, or sequential bilateral thoracotomies. However, with the widespread acceptance of video-assisted thoracic surgery (VATS) for the treatment of primary lung conditions, many surgeons have challenged the need for open approaches to pulmonary metastasectomy.

Thoracoscopic pulmonary resection has been shown to have several potential advantages over open approaches. VATS has been shown to minimize the immunologic impact of surgery with reduced proinflammatory cytokines and measurably increased endogenous antitumor natural killer cells compared with thoracotomy.[6–8] The effect of this immunologic milieu on the patient with cancer remains unproven; however, the theoretic benefit may be particularly relevant in the patient with metastatic disease given increasing evidence for important immune escape mechanisms in cancer metastasis.[9,10] In addition, results from the Cancer and Leukemia Group B (CALGB) 31,001 study published in 2015 have demonstrated VATS lobectomy to have shorter length of hospital stay and decreased perioperative complications compared with open surgery.[11]

Ensuring speedy recovery and minimizing systemic insult is a priority in patients with metastatic disease, as surgery will frequently be coupled with systemic therapy and undue delays can result from prolonged hospitalization and deconditioning.

The lung is the most common site of relapse after pulmonary metastasectomy, for both epithelial cancers and sarcoma.[12,13] In 1998, an Austrian study including 330 patients who underwent 2 or more resections for lung metastases demonstrated the feasibility and safety of repeat metastasectomy in appropriately chosen patients. Similarly, Jaklitsch and colleagues[14] demonstrated that repeat pulmonary metastasectomy can reestablish local control and provides survival benefit even after multiple recurrences, albeit with somewhat diminishing returns after each subsequent operation. These data support a practice of surgical resection for recurrent lung metastases, which can be predicted to occur in as many as 53% of patients based on the data of Pastorino and colleagues.[3] Therefore, given the reasonable likelihood of recurrence, the decreased adhesion formation and potentially easier repeat operation after thoracoscopic metastasectomy, a minimally invasive approach may be preferred.[15] Furthermore, the ability to successfully perform repeat metastasectomy calls into question the benefit of mandatory bimanual palpation to identify lesions below the threshold of computed tomography (CT) scan detection if, in fact, these lesions can be successfully addressed in a subsequent operation once detected by surveillance imaging.

Critics frequently object to the reliance on preoperative imaging to direct resection in thoracoscopic pulmonary metastasectomy. Opponents voice concerns that thoracoscopy leads to missed lesions at metastasectomy and only with open thoracotomy can one rest assured that every nodule is found and removed. However, current CT scanners can detect nodules as small as 2 to 3 mm, and resolution continues to improve. With modern imaging technology, we are identifying lesions that may be difficult to palpate even using an open bimanual technique. The aforementioned data from the Brigham and Women's Hospital[14] suggest that leaving nodules behind that fall below this size threshold may not be as clinically significant as once assumed. The metastasectomy patient will be monitored in a close follow-up surveillance program and pulmonary metastases (new or missed) will be recognized as soon as they reach the imaging threshold. In this strategy, the goal of metastasectomy is to remove all known lesions based on preoperative imaging and not necessarily an exhaustive search for otherwise unidentified nodules. Following this protocol does not appear to deleteriously affect survival; however, this has not been tested in a prospective randomized fashion.

Taken together, the data suggest several benefits to thoracoscopic pulmonary metastasectomy. In the ensuing section we describe our standard VATS technique, which represents our preferred operative strategy for pulmonary metastasectomy.

SURGICAL TECHNIQUE
Preoperative Planning

Preoperative preparation for thoracoscopic pulmonary metastasectomy mirrors that which is performed for any thoracoscopic lung resection. A CT scan of the chest is considered mandatory and ideally performed within 4 weeks of the operation.[16] Importantly, additional studies to complete the metastatic workup should have been performed to ensure the absence of occult distant disease, including PET/CT or brain MRI, depending on the stage and histology of the primary tumor. Pulmonary function tests are performed, spirometry and diffusion, to evaluate respiratory reserve. Additional cardiopulmonary testing, such as transthoracic echocardiogram, cardiac stress testing, and/or cardiac catheterization are obtained on an individual case basis. Patients should be counseled that conversion to thoracotomy may be required to achieve the goal of complete removal of all lesions detected by preoperative CT scan; however, small lesions below the threshold of detection could be left behind. A frank discussion regarding the chance of pulmonary recurrence should occur preoperatively, including the possibility of repeat metastasectomy. Most importantly, meticulous review of the preoperative cross-sectional imaging is imperative before embarking on thoracoscopic metastasectomy.

Each surgeon must recognize the importance of translating the 2-dimensional images of a high-quality CT scan to the 3-dimensional chest anatomy and, more specifically, the topography of the lung. We make a practice of dividing the chest into thirds from superior to inferior: above the azygous/aortic arch, between the azygous/aortic arch and the inferior pulmonary vein, and below the inferior pulmonary vein. Next these thirds are subdivided into thirds by the anterior and posterior axillary lines; effectively dividing the hemithorax into a 3 × 3 matrix. This method in combination with a thorough working knowledge of the segmental pulmonary anatomy allows for identification of each lesion seen on preoperative imaging. Whatever method one uses, the ability to reliably identify all lesions seen on CT scan using the thoracoscope without bimanual palpation is the key to VATS metastasectomy.

Preparation and Patient Positioning

Thoracoscopic metastasectomy requires excellent single-lung isolation. Complete collapse of the lung facilitates palpation of intraparenchymal nodules using thoracoscopic instruments or by the surgeon's finger through working ports. Lung isolation also allows for better visualization of certain surface irregularities suggestive of an underlying abnormality (puckering, discoloration, or bulging). Single-lung ventilation is achieved by using either a bronchial blocker or double-lumen endotracheal tube.

The patient is positioned in full lateral decubitus position with all pressure points adequately protected. We find that flexion of the bed is typically

not required with the exception of patients having particularly prominent iliac crests. In such cases, slight flexion of the bed can drop the angle between the hip and the chest wall allowing for improved mobility of the thoracoscope.

Surgical Approach

Several techniques have been reported for thoracoscopic lung resection. Methods include 2 to 4 ports with or without a utility incision, hybrid approach combining VATS and open techniques,[17] robotic-assisted,[18] and more recently, uniportal approaches.[19,20] Regardless of approach, the principles of avoiding rib spreading, protection of the intercostal bundle, and identification of the target lesion remain constant. We generally use a 3-incision technique with an inferior camera port, a posterior working port, and an anterior working port that can be extended to a utility incision (**Fig. 1**). In cases with a high likelihood of conversion to open thoracotomy, the VATS incisions should be planned in such a way that at least one can be incorporated into the anticipated thoracotomy incision.

Surgical Procedure

We start by placing the inferior camera port once the anesthesiologist has isolated the ipsilateral lung. The camera port is placed in the seventh or

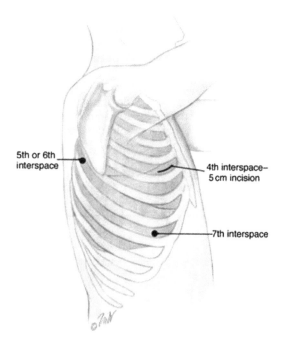

5th or 6th interspace

4th interspace– 5 cm incision

7th interspace

Fig. 1. Three-incision technique. (*From* Sugarbaker DJ, Bueno R, Krasna MJ, et al, editors. Adult chest surgery. New York: McGraw-Hill; 2009; with permission.)

eighth intercostal space, the specific location of which depends on the target lesions and diaphragm location based on careful review of preoperative imaging. Use of a 30-degree thoracoscope provides a superior view allowing the surgeon to see around corners and avoiding crowding instruments and struggling against the camera. Oftentimes the lesion of interest can be identified using solely the camera port with a narrow dissecting instrument, such as the endoscopic Kittner, placed beside the camera. In this manner, the additional working ports can be placed to precisely triangulate the lesion of interest for simultaneous grasping and lifting of the lesions through one port and endoscopic stapler placement through the other working port (**Fig. 2**). In the event that the target lesion or lesions cannot be readily identified, the additional working ports are placed with attention to the anticipated locations of the targets based on imaging. Next the surgeon sequentially grasps and lifts lung tissue from the posterior port and inserts a ring clamp (or a finger) via the anterior port for palpation. An underlying lesion can be seen and felt to bounce off the clamp as it passes over. Using these techniques, we are most often able to identify all lesions seen on CT scan without needing to convert to an open incision.

Once the metastatic nodule has been located, the tissue is excised with a goal 1-cm margin of normal lung using endoscopic stapling devices. We typically use the medium tissue thickness staple cartridge on lung parenchyma allowing for adequate tissue compression before stapling as directed by the manufacturer. In the event that the nodule or mass is located centrally or in close proximity to a named vessel or bronchus, a sublobar wedge resection may not provide an adequate tissue margin. In these cases, we perform anatomic segmentectomy or lobectomy with careful consideration of the

patient's pulmonary function. Lung preservation is a primary goal in these patients, as optimizing quality of life is a priority and recurrence is possible. Furthermore, optimizing pulmonary reserve and recovery will facilitate successfully providing adjuvant chemotherapy in appropriate patients.

Following metastasectomy, we place a pleural drainage tube via the prior camera port. We also routinely perform intercostal nerve blocks using bupivacaine. The lung parenchyma is reinflated under direct thoracoscopic vision to ensure adequate inflation, no torsion, and proper positioning of the chest tube. Patients are extubated before leaving the operating room and recovered in the postanesthesia care unit (PACU) before a short stay in the thoracic intermediate care floor unit.

REHABILITATION AND RECOVERY

The postoperative course following thoracoscopic pulmonary metastasectomy is typically amenable to a "fast-track" protocol. In lieu of significant air leak, chest drains can be placed to water seal in the PACU. We find most chest drains can be removed promptly the following morning during rounds based on clinical criteria (eg, low output, no air leak) without first requiring a chest radiograph. Pain is controlled with oral narcotics and, assuming no contraindications, nonsteroidal anti-inflammatory drugs, such as intravenous ketorolac, which is converted to oral ibuprofen once the patient has demonstrated tolerance of oral intake. We do not typical use epidural catheters for patients undergoing VATS procedures unless preoperative evaluation suggests a high likely of conversion to thoracotomy. As is standard for all patients following lung resection, we encourage early ambulation and pulmonary toilet exercises beginning immediately after surgery. Most

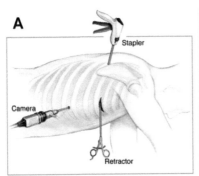
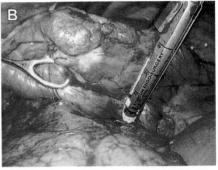

Fig. 2. The additional working ports can be placed to precisely triangulate the lesion of interest for simultaneous grasping and lifting of the lesions through one port and endoscopic stapler placement through the other working port. (*A*) Port Placement. (*B*) Picture of lung being grasped and resected with stapler. (*From* Sugarbaker DJ, Bueno R, Krasna MJ, et al, editors. Adult chest surgery. New York: McGraw-Hill; 2009; with permission.)

patients are able to leave the hospital on the first postoperative day.

CLINICAL RESULTS IN THE LITERATURE

The controversy surrounding pulmonary metastasectomy is compounded by a lack of prospective, randomized data. To date, there has been no trial to evaluate the survival advantage of pulmonary metastasectomy compared with nonoperative management. Similarly, there is no randomized comparison of the minimally invasive thoracoscopic approach to standard open techniques for metastatic disease to the lungs. Nevertheless, several investigators have described their experiences with VATS versus open pulmonary metastasectomy and we describe these data in the ensuing section.

The concept of missed lesions during thoracoscopy has been the focus of several studies. In 2009, Cerfolio and colleagues[21] published an analysis of 57 patients who underwent thoracotomy for metastatic pulmonary disease, but retrospectively met criteria for thoracoscopic resection. In 21 of the 57 patients, bimanual palpation identified nodules that were not detected by preoperative 64-slice helical CT scan. However, in only 10 of these 21 patients were the missed nodules malignant on final pathologic evaluation. In other words, in this study, bimanual palpation led to the resection of additional benign nodules in 19.3% of patients. In a more recent study, Eckardt and colleagues[22] performed a prospective blinded evaluation of thoracoscopic versus open metastasectomy. In this study, one surgical team performed thoracoscopic metastasectomy followed by a second team that performed thoracotomy on the same patient. Thoracoscopy identified 87% of the 140 nodules in 89 patients who were seen on preoperative CT scan. However, thoracotomy identified an additional 67 nodules of which 22 (33%) were metastatic lesions. The investigators, therefore, conclude that VATS metastasectomy is inadequate if one assumes the goal of surgery is to resect all pulmonary nodules. Collectively, these studies demonstrate that bimanual palpation during open thoracotomy may detect small lesions that are missed by even modern CT scanning and thoracoscopic evaluation. However, whether these missed nodules affect oncologic outcome in terms of overall or disease-specific survival cannot be determined from these reports.

One the first studies to compare outcomes of thoracoscopic metastasectomy with open thoracotomy was published in 2002 by Mutsaerts and colleagues.[23] This group from the Netherlands compared 19 patients undergoing VATS with 16 patients having confirmatory thoracotomy. Complications were higher in the thoracotomy group (5 vs 0, $P = .049$) and 2-year overall survival was similar (70% vs 67%). It is notable that only patients with solitary, peripheral lesions smaller than 3 cm were included in this analysis. The investigators concluded that in this subset of patients, thoracoscopic resection is at least oncologically comparable to an open operation. In 2008, Nakajima and colleagues[24] published a substantially larger retrospective cohort study comparing 72 patients who underwent VATS with 71 patients having had thoracotomy for colorectal pulmonary metastases. In this Japanese study, 5-year recurrence-free survival was improved in the thoracoscopic group (34.4% vs 21.1%, $P = .047$) and there was no difference in overall survival (49.3% vs 39.5%). The investigators concluded that thoracoscopic metastasectomy was justified in the setting of pulmonary metastases from colorectal cancer. Similarly supportive results were reported for sarcoma metastases by Gossot and colleagues[25] in 2009. The French group compared 31 patients undergoing VATS resection with 29 undergoing thoracotomy, but who on retrospective review had preoperative characteristics that would have allowed for a VATS approach. To be included in the analysis, patients needed to have 2 or fewer metastases each of which could be no larger than 3 cm and only wedge resections were included. One-year, 3-year, and 5-year overall survival ($P = .2$), as well as 1-year and 3-year disease-free survival ($P = .74$) were similar between the VATS and thoracotomy groups. However, postoperative length of stay was 3.7 days after thoracoscopic resection and 6.2 days after thoracotomy ($P<.0001$). The investigators suggested that the decreased length of stay and preserving the ability to undergo repeat metastasectomy were important benefits of the thoracoscopic approach. Finally, another 2009 retrospective study by Carballo and colleagues[26] found equivalent 5-year recurrence-free survival comparing 135 patients treated with thoracotomy with 36 patients having VATS resection for pulmonary metastases from primaries of mixed histologies (51% vs 67%, $P = .27$).

The major limitation of these retrospective studies is an inherent patient selection bias. Nevertheless, these studies suggest thoracoscopic metastasectomy can be performed safely and, in appropriately selected patients, yields at least equivalent survival compared with open thoracotomy. A prospective randomized trial is needed to truly decipher the relative risks and benefits of the thoracoscopic approach, as well as the consequence of missed lesions after thoracoscopic metastasectomy.

Additional controversy surrounds the role for mediastinal lymph node dissection in the setting of pulmonary metastasectomy. Some investigators have suggested that thoracotomy can achieve an improved lymphadenectomy and is a reason to avoid thoracoscopic pulmonary metastasectomy.[25] A 2008 survey of members of the European Society of Thoracic Surgery revealed that 55% of surgeons performed some degree of mediastinal lymph node sampling during the course of metastasectomy, whereas 33% of respondents never perform nodal dissection; thus, highlighting the lack of a clearly defined standard.[27] However, there is an increasing body of literature supporting the role of lymphadenectomy for pulmonary metastasectomy. In 2001, Loehe and colleagues[28] studied 71 pulmonary metastasectomies in 63 patients and found a 14.3% incidence of unexpected nodal disease unrecognized by preoperative CT scan, a number comparable to that in non–small cell lung cancer wherein mediastinal lymph node evaluation is considered standard of care. The investigators also reported a trend toward improved survival in patients without nodal involvement and concluded that nodal dissection should be performed routinely in these patients. Similarly, a study by Pfannschmidt and colleagues[29] retrospectively analyzed 245 patients undergoing pulmonary metastasectomy for hilar and mediastinal lymph node involvement. Median survival was significantly improved in patents determined to be pN0 compared with pN1 ($P = .018$) and pN2 ($P = .001$). The article concludes that routine nodal dissection during metastasectomy may improve prognostication and aid in individualized decisions regarding adjuvant therapies. Notably, no data are included regarding complications related to the additional node dissection. The patients included in these studies underwent thoracotomy; however, there are several studies supporting the efficacy of thoracoscopic lymph node dissection. D'Amico and colleagues[30] published an analysis of 4215 patients from the National Comprehensive Cancer Network database comparing the efficacy of thoracoscopic versus open mediastinal lymph node dissection in the setting of lobectomy for lung cancer. Lymphadenectomy was equivalent with respect to number of nodes and nodal stations dissected. Similar results were found in a smaller prospective randomized trial published in 2013 by Palade and colleagues[31] comparing thoracoscopic (n = 34) versus open (n = 32) mediastinal lymph node dissection in early-stage lung cancer. Taken together, these data suggest that there may be a prognostic role for lymph node dissection during pulmonary metastasectomy in tumors with known predilection for lymphatic involvement and that thoracoscopic lymphadenectomy is a safe and efficacious surgical approach.

SUMMARY

Although no prospective, randomized trials exist, the preponderance of data support pulmonary metastasectomy in appropriately selected patients.[32] These patients will frequently require multimodality therapy, including systemic chemotherapy and/or immunotherapy to address the totality of their disease. In this setting, there must be a carefully planned balance between the oncologic priority of complete disease eradication and the equally important goal of minimizing pain, hospitalization, and delay of adjuvant therapies. Thoracoscopic resection appears to achieve these goals by reducing immunologic insult, postoperative complications, and hospital length of stay, thereby providing these patients an optimal surgical recovery and quality of life in an otherwise emotionally and physically taxing time. Concerns regarding the inability to palpate the entire lung and reliance on preoperative imaging appear to be overemphasized given the improving sensitivity of spiral chest CT scanning, the efficacy of repeat metastasectomy, and the unclear clinical significance of lesions smaller than the size threshold of detection. Standard VATS techniques are applicable to pulmonary metastasectomy with the primary goal of excising all lesions seen on preoperative cross-sectional imaging. To this end, although several investigators have argued that open metastasectomy can identify additional occult lesions not seen on CT scan compared with thoracoscopy, this has never been shown to impact survival. In addition, certain histologies may benefit from concomitant lymph node dissection during pulmonary metastasectomy, which can be performed using VATS techniques. We support thoracoscopic pulmonary metastasectomy as first-line surgical therapy in appropriately selected patients, followed by aggressive CT scan surveillance, and repeat thoracoscopic metastasectomy for recurrent lung metastases.

REFERENCES

1. Barney JJ. A twelve-year cure following nephrectomy for adenocarcinoma and lobectomy for solitary metastasis. Trans Am Assoc Genitourin Surg 1945; 37:189–91.
2. Aberg T, Malmberg KA, Nilsson B, et al. The effect of metastasectomy: fact or fiction? Ann Thorac Surg 1980;30:378–84.
3. Pastorino U, Buyse M, Friedel G, et al. Long-term results of lung metastasectomy: prognostic analyses

based on 5206 cases. J Thorac Cardiovasc Surg 1997;113:37–49.

4. Margaritora S, Porziella V, D'Andrilli A, et al. Pulmonary metastases: can accurate radiological evaluation avoid thoracotomic approach? Eur J Cardiothoracic Surg 2002;21:1111–4.

5. Parsons AM, Detterbeck FC, Parker LA. Accuracy of helical CT in the detection of pulmonary metastases: is intraoperative palpation still necessary? Ann Thorac Surg 2004;78:1910–6 [discussion: 6–8].

6. Ng CS, Wan S, Hui CW, et al. Video-assisted thoracic surgery for early stage lung cancer—can short-term immunological advantages improve long-term survival? Ann Thorac Cardiovasc Surg 2006;12:308–12.

7. Yim AP, Wan S, Lee TW, et al. VATS lobectomy reduces cytokine responses compared with conventional surgery. Ann Thorac Surg 2000;70:243–7.

8. McKenna RJ, Mahtabifard A, Swanson SJ. Atlas of minimally invasive thoracic surgery (VATS). 1st edition. Philadelphia: Elsevier/Saunders; 2011.

9. Croci DO, Salatino M. Tumor immune escape mechanisms that operate during metastasis. Curr Pharm Biotechnol 2011;12:1923–36.

10. Pancione M, Giordano G, Remo A, et al. Immune escape mechanisms in colorectal cancer pathogenesis and liver metastasis. J Immunol Res 2014;2014: 686879.

11. Nwogu CE, D'Cunha J, Pang H, et al. VATS lobectomy has better perioperative outcomes than open lobectomy: CALGB 31001, an ancillary analysis of CALGB 140202 (Alliance). Ann Thorac Surg 2015; 99:399–405.

12. Monteiro A, Arce N, Bernardo J, et al. Surgical resection of lung metastases from epithelial tumors. Ann Thorac Surg 2004;77:431–7.

13. Temple LK, Brennan MF. The role of pulmonary metastasectomy in soft tissue sarcoma. Semin Thorac Cardiovasc Surg 2002;14:35–44.

14. Jaklitsch MT, Mery CM, Lukanich JM, et al. Sequential thoracic metastasectomy prolongs survival by re-establishing local control within the chest. J Thorac Cardiovasc Surg 2001;121:657–67.

15. Tanaka K, Hida Y, Kaga K, et al. Video-assisted thoracoscopic surgery lowers the incidence of adhesion to the chest wall but not to the mediastinal and interlobar pleurae. Surg Laparosc Endosc Percutan Tech 2010;20:46–8.

16. Detterbeck FC, Grodzki T, Gleeson F, et al. Imaging requirements in the practice of pulmonary metastasectomy. J Thorac Oncol 2010;5:S134–9.

17. Raza A, Takabe K, Wolfe LG, et al. Outcomes of hybrid video assisted thoracoscopic surgery for pulmonary metastasectomy. J Surg Sci 2014;2:18–24.

18. Wei B, D'Amico TA. Thoracoscopic versus robotic approaches: advantages and disadvantages. Thorac Surg Clin 2014;24:177–88.

19. Hung MH, Cheng YJ, Chan KC, et al. Nonintubated uniportal thoracoscopic surgery for peripheral lung nodules. Ann Thorac Surg 2014;98:1998–2003.

20. Song IH, Yum S, Choi W, et al. Clinical application of single incision thoracoscopic surgery: early experience of 264 cases. J Cardiothorac Surg 2014;9:44.

21. Cerfolio RJ, McCarty T, Bryant AS. Non-Imaged Pulmonary Nodules Discovered During Thoracotomy for Metastasectomy by Lung Palpation. Eur J CardioTorac Surg 2009;35(5):786–91.

22. Eckhardt J, Licht PB. Thoracoscopic or Open Surgery for Pulmonary Metastasectomy: An Observer Blinded Study. Ann Thorac Surg 2014;98(2):466–9.

23. Mutsaerts EL, Zoetmulder FA, Meijer S, et al. Long term survival of thoracoscopic metastasectomy vs metastasectomy by thoracotomy in patients with a solitary pulmonary lesion. Eur J Surg Oncol 2002; 28:864–8.

24. Nakajima J, Murakawa T, Fukami T, et al. Is thoracoscopic surgery justified to treat pulmonary metastasis from colorectal cancer? Interact Cardiovasc Thorac Surg 2008;7:212–6 [discussion: 6–7].

25. Gossot D, Radu C, Girard P, et al. Resection of pulmonary metastases from sarcoma: can some patients benefit from a less invasive approach? Ann Thorac Surg 2009;87:238–43.

26. Carballo M, Maish MS, Jaroszewski DE, et al. Video-assisted thoracic surgery (VATS) as a safe alternative for the resection of pulmonary metastases: a retrospective cohort study. J Cardiothorac Surg 2009;4:13.

27. Internullo E, Cassivi SD, Van Raemdonck D, et al, ESTS Pulmonary Metastasectomy Working Group. Pulmonary metastasectomy: a survey of current practice amongst members of the European Society of Thoracic Surgeons. J Thorac Oncol 2008;3: 1257–66.

28. Loehe F, Kobinger S, Hatz RA, et al. Value of systematic mediastinal lymph node dissection during pulmonary metastasectomy. Ann Thorac Surg 2001; 72:225–9.

29. Pfannschmidt J, Klode J, Muley T, et al. Nodal involvement at the time of pulmonary metastasectomy: experiences in 245 patients. Ann Thorac Surg 2006;81:448–54.

30. D'Amico TA, Niland J, Mamet R, et al. Efficacy of mediastinal lymph node dissection during lobectomy for lung cancer by thoracoscopy and thoracotomy. Ann Thorac Surg 2011;92:226–31 [discussion: 31–2].

31. Palade E, Passlick B, Osei-Agyemang T, et al. Video-assisted vs open mediastinal lymphadenectomy for stage I non-small-cell lung cancer: results of a prospective randomized trial. Eur J Cardiothoracic Surg 2013;44:244–9 [discussion: 9].

32. Erhunmwunsee L, D'Amico TA. Surgical management of pulmonary metastases. Ann Thorac Surg 2009;88:2052–60.

Results of Pulmonary Resection
Other Epithelial Malignancies

Stefan Sponholz, MD, Moritz Schirren, MD, Natalie Kudelin, MD,
Elisabeth Knöchlein, MD, Joachim Schirren, MD*

KEYWORDS

- Breast cancer • Renal cell cancer • Metastasectomy • Lymphadenectomy • Lung metastases

KEY POINTS

- Detected pulmonary nodules in patients with breast cancer represent a second cancer in up to 60% of cases (usually lung cancer).
- For selected patients, a combination of systemic therapy and surgery is reasonable.
- The role of systemic therapy after metastasectomy in patients with oligometastases and long disease-free interval must be evaluated in the future.
- Complete resection of lung metastases from renal cell cancer in selected patients is the therapy of choice.
- Systematic lymph node dissection during pulmonary metastasectomy of renal cell cancer should be considered.

THE ROLE OF METASTASECTOMY IN PATIENTS WITH BREAST CANCER

Breast cancer is the second most common cancer worldwide. It is the most common for women, with 1.67 million cases diagnosed in 2012. Compared with other tumor entities, it is fifth in cases of death.[1] The 5-year survival rate is between 22% and 100%.[2] In the first 5 years, the tumor recurs in 30% of the patients. In these cases, up to 36% are a local recurrence, up to 58% a distant recurrence, and up to 6% a local and distant recurrence.[3] The incidence of lung metastases in patients with breast cancer is between 7% and 24%, and they are most common in HER2-positive and basal-like histologies.[4] The spectrum of therapy for metastatic breast cancer may include chemotherapy, targeted anti-HER2 therapy, hormonal therapy, surgical treatment, and radiation. Adjuvant and neoadjuvant treatment is now patient customized with better survival rates, even in overall survival (OS) or in progression free survival.[5]

Regarding the resection of lung metastases from breast cancer, there is no consensus found in the literature, but therapy may include chemotherapy followed by metastasectomy.[6] In our clinic, an observation period of at least 2 months from first diagnosed lung metastases is used. During this time, we can evaluate the dynamics of the disease, including the development of new pulmonary metastases or the development of extrapulmonary metastases. In general, the indications for operation are:

- Solitary nodules after treatment
- Residual nodule after chemotherapy
- Resectable metastatic recurrences

There is no commercial or financial conflict of interest or funding sources.
Department of Thoracic Surgery, Dr Horst Schmidt Klinik, Ludwig-Erhard-Strasse 100, Wiesbaden 65199, Germany
* Corresponding author.
E-mail address: joachim.schirren@helios-kliniken.de

Thorac Surg Clin 26 (2016) 99–108
http://dx.doi.org/10.1016/j.thorsurg.2015.09.012

Furthermore, there are palliative indications for metastasectomy:

- Tumor erosion into the airways with hemorrhage or septic complications
- Infiltration of the chest wall
- Therapy-resistant pleural effusion.[7]

Generally, prerequisites for operation are:

- Local control of primary tumor
- No extrapulmonary metastases (with possible exceptions)
- No alternative treatment available
- Resectability of all metastases
- Justifiable general and functional risks[7]

The final decision for an operative treatment should be made by an interdisciplinary tumor board that includes thoracic surgeons, oncologists, gynecologists, radiotherapists, and radiologists.

DIAGNOSIS

The European Society for Medical Oncology guidelines for breast cancer do not recommend a thoracic imaging in the follow-up of initial breast cancer therapy.[8] However, Singletary and colleagues[9] recommended that a chest radiograph should be part of the follow-up to detect early lung nodules, and computed tomography (CT) is most commonly used to evaluate lung metastases.[10] In addition fluorodeoxyglucose PET (FDG-PET), alone or in combination with CT (FDG-PET/CT), improves the ability to assess for intrathoracic and extrathoracic metastases and to evaluate the response to medical treatment.[11] MRI is reserved for patients with locally invasive chest wall lesions.[12,13] Despite all radiological techniques Vogt-Moykopf and colleagues[7] showed that only 39% of the preoperatively diagnosed number of metastases corresponds to the postoperative number of metastases. They showed that palpation of the lung is the most sensitive procedure for detecting lung metastases.[7] Cerfolio and colleagues[13] confirmed this conclusion fifteen years later. They resected suspected nodules per thoracotomy, which normally could be resected by thoracoscopy. In their results they found 37% nodules, which were not seen by imaging and 48% of them were metastases.[13]

LUNG CANCER VERSUS METASTASIS BREAST CANCER

If a solitary pulmonary nodule is detected in a patient with breast cancer, in approximately 60% of cases it represents a second primary cancer (usually lung cancer), in about 30% it represents metastasis of the breast cancer, and in 10% it is benign.[14] For this reason it is essential to prove the histology before metastasectomy when possible. It can also be very difficult for the pathologist to differentiate between a breast cancer and a lung cancer in the intraoperative frozen section, especially for adenocarcinomas.

A fine-needle biopsy to get tissue can be done by bronchoscopy (central nodule) or CT (peripheral). Additionally, a video-assisted thoracoscopy can help determine if the nodule is reachable. If it is not reachable, a thoracotomy with intraoperative frozen section can be an option.[15]

In addition to the diagnosis of pulmonary nodules, lymph node involvement plays an important role. One fourth of the patients with resected lung metastases from breast cancer have lymph node metastases.[6,16] The cause might be the central location of the lung metastases and the direct pathway through lymph vessels. This differs for the primary tumor entities (**Figs. 1** and **2**).

In cases of lymph node metastases of breast cancer especially, FDG-PET and PET/CT are more sensitive than CT of the chest.[11]

SURVIVAL

The role of pulmonary metastasectomy in patients with breast cancer is patient specific, depending on the use and response to previous treatment, receptor status of the primary tumor, and other factors. This decision should be made for every patient by a multidisciplinary tumor board.

The first resection of a pulmonary metastasis from breast cancer was in 1921 by Röpke.[17] Yoshimoto and colleagues[18] reviewed the survival of their patients with breast cancer metastases after metastasectomy from 1960 to 2000. The 5-year survival rate was 54%, and the 10-year survival rate was 40%, with a median survival of 6.3 years. The 5-year survival rate in the studies before 2000 ranges from 31% to 62% with a median survival between 33 and 54 months.[7,19–22] After 2000, the

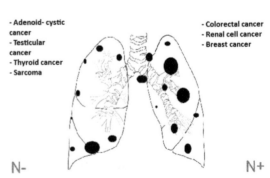

Fig. 1. Metastatic spread of different tumor entities.

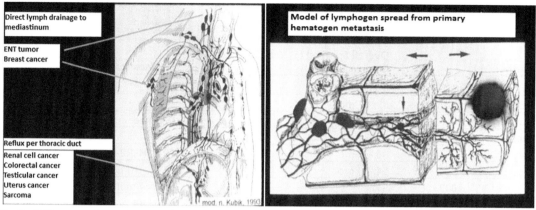

Fig. 2. Different path mechanism of lymph node metastases. ENT, ear, nose throat.

5-year survival rate ranges between 31% and 54% with a median survival between 32 and 97 months[16,18,23–28] (**Tables 1** and **2**). This analysis shows that resection for lung metastases from breast cancer is associated with acceptable overall survival in selected patients.

In a study by Staren and colleagues,[20] there was a significant difference between patients with only systemic therapy and patients with added surgical therapy (33 vs 55 months). There was no positive influence in OS for chemotherapy before or after resection of lung metastases in the study by Friedel and colleagues.[23] For patients without chemotherapy treatment, the 5-year survival rate was 39%, with chemotherapy before metastasectomy 20% and after resection 44%. Patients receiving chemotherapy before and after the resection survived fewer than 5 years. The study could not account for selection bias; however, as patients with more advanced disease were more likely to receive chemotherapy. Nevertheless, the study shows that some patients with only surgical resection can achieve a good OS. Yhim and colleagues[29] compared outcomes of the combination of resection and systemic therapy or only systemic therapy in patients with fewer than 4 pulmonary metastases. The patients with the combination had a 4-year survival rate of 82% compared with a 4-year survival rate of 32% for the patients without resection ($P = .001$).

More trials are necessary, especially ones with prospective study design, to investigate more precisely the effect of pulmonary metastasectomy from breast cancer and the relative roles of surgery and systemic therapy.

PROGNOSTIC FACTORS

Several prognostic indicators for selecting patients for pulmonary metastasectomy have been studied, for all primary histologies, including disease-free interval (interval between original diagnosis of the primary and the development of pulmonary metastases), complete resection, number of nodules, and other biologic factors. In the existing literature, several studies define a long

| Table 1 |
| Publications of pulmonary metastasectomy from breast cancer before 2000 |

Author, Year	Overall Survival (5- Year Survival [%]; Median Survival)	Prognosticators
Lanza et al,[19] 1992	50; 47 mo	DFI, (ER+)
Staren et al,[20] 1992	36; 54 mo	—
Vogt-Moykopf et al,[7] 1994	31; 33 mo	DFI, LNM-, <2 met
McDonald et al,[21] 1994	38; 42 mo	—
Simpson et al,[22] 1997	62	—

Abbreviations: ER+, estrogen receptor; HER2+, HER2 receptor; met, metastases.

Table 2
Publications of pulmonary metastasectomy from breast cancer after 2000

Author, Year	Overall Survival (5- Year Survival [%]; Median Survival)	Prognosticators
Friedel et al,[23] 2002	35; 35 mo	DFI, R0
Ludwig et al,[24] 2003	53; 97 mo	DFI
Planchard et al,[25] 2004	45; 50 mo	DFI, size
Tanaka et al,[26] 2005	31; 32 mo	—
Welter et al,[16] 2008	36; 32 mo	ER+, HER2+
Yoshimoto et al,[18] 2008	54; 76 mo	DFI
Chen et al,[27] 2009	51	DFI, <4 met
Yhim et al,[29] 2010	82 (4y and only <4 met)	DFI, ER+
Meimarakis et al,[28] 2013	82 mo	ER+, HER2+, R0, size, <2, (LNM)

Abbreviations: ER+, estrogen receptor; HER2+, HER2 receptor; met, metastases; R0, complete resection; size, size of metastasis.

disease-free interval (DFI) as a significant prognostic factor for a longer OS. The specific DFI used as a prognostic indicator varies among studies between 12 months and 42 months.[7,18,19,23–25,27,29] Most of the studies choose a DFI of 3 years.[18,23,25,27]

Complete resection is found to be the most important prognostic indicator for most primary histologies, although its relation to biology of the tumor and tumor burden is intertwined. Friedel and colleagues[23] showed, at complete resection, a 5-year survival rate of 38%, a 10-year survival rate of 22%, and a 15-year survival rate of 20%. Patients with incomplete resection had a 5-year survival rate of 18% and survived less than 10 years. The number of metastases is also a controversial topic. In their study, Vogt-Moykopf and collogues[7] found an obvious difference between single and multiple metastases (5-year 44% vs 14%), a finding replicated in other studies[27,28] but not in all studies.[23–25] A distinctive characteristic of breast cancer is the role of hormone receptors for treatment and prognosis.[16,19,28,29] Welter and colleagues[16] found a 5-year survival rate for patients with positive estrogen receptor status of 77% (vs 12% if negative) and for patients with positive HER2 status of 74% (vs 22% if negative). However, an adjuvant hormonal treatment was also associated with less tumor progression compared with chemotherapy, which could explain the prolonged survival. The possibility that the status of the receptor can vary between the primary and the metastasis is known.[30] For this reason, tissue acquisition from the metastasis to identify the receptor status is advantageous.

The prognostic influence of the presence of lymph node metastases (LNM) is controversial.

According to Vogt-Moykopf and collogues,[7] no patient with LNM reached the 5-year survival mark. Patients without LNM had a 5-year survival rate of 38%. This finding is confirmed by some investigators[28] but not by all.[24,25]

PROGNOSTIC GROUPS

The use of prognostic group stratification may improve the ability to select patients for resection. Prognostic groups may be classified in patients without risk factors (group 1), only 1 risk factor (group 2), 2 risk factors (group 3), and unresectable patients (group 4). The risk factors under consideration are DFI less than 36 months and multiple metastases. Group 1 had a 5-year survival rate of 50%, a 10-year survival rate of 26%, and a 15-year survival rate of 26%. Group 2 also had a promising 5-year survival rate of 35%, a 10-year survival rate of 21%, and a 15-year survival rate of 18%. Only groups 3 and 4 did not benefit from resection.[23]

For selected patients, we currently consider a combination of systemic therapy and surgery in terms of a residual tumor resection reasonable. Furthermore, the role of systemic therapy after metastasectomy in patients with singular metastasis and long DFI must be evaluated in the future.

THE ROLE OF METASTASECTOMY IN PATIENTS WITH RENAL CELL CANCER

Renal cell cancer (RCC) is the 12th most common cancer and the 16th most common cause of death by cancer worldwide,[1] and In 2012, 338,000 new cases were diagnosed.[31] After resection of the primary tumor, local recurrence is rare, but 20% to 30% of patients subsequently have distant recurrence. Lung metastases are the most common (up to 60%).[32] The rate for synchronous lung metastases is between 17% and 40%. Most patients have multiple metastases.[33,34] The use of adjuvant therapy after resection of the primary tumor is currently not established.[35]

Because of its resistance to chemotherapy, metastatic RCC is a challenge to treat. Therapeutic regimens with cytokines result in partial response in only 15% to 20% of patients. Newer therapies with tyrosine kinase inhibitors are showing better response, up to 40%, but a complete remission is rarely reached.[35,36] Nevertheless, for selected patients, resection of lung metastases with mediastinal lymph node dissection is associated with long-term survival.[6,7,37-41] For patients that are not candidates for resection, stereotactic radiation has been used for those with up to 3 metastases, with local control achieved in 90% to 98% of patients.[42]

DIAGNOSIS

For the detection of lung metastases of RCC, CT is considered to be the gold standard. The *National Comprehensive Cancer Network* guidelines recommend, after a nephrectomy of stage I tumors, an annual CT in the first 3 years and, if necessary, even after this period. After radical nephrectomy of stage II and III cancers, CT is recommended in the first 3 to 6 months and should be followed at this interval for 3 years. After this period, it should be conducted annually for 5 years.[43]

For the primary cancer, PET/CT plays a minor role, but for detection of metastases it has a good rate of sensitivity between 87% and 89% and a good rate of specificity between 83% and 93%.[44-46] In addition, studies are currently being conducted to determine if PET/CT can evaluate the response of tyrosine kinase inhibitors.[47]

As with other tumor entities, it is necessary to exclude extrathoracic metastases and an infiltration of centrally located structures with common diagnoses.

Winter and colleagues[48] found a higher sensitivity and specificity for detecting mediastinal lymph node involvement (90% and 97%) than for hilar lymph node metastases (69% and 87%) per CT. For both, the sensitivity was 84% and the specificity was 97%. Pastorino and colleagues[46] were able to find an advantage for staging of lymph node metastases by PET/CT compared with CT. The sensitivity for resected patients was 87%.

SURVIVAL

Barney and Churchill[49] were the first to publish their results in 1939 for the resection of a lung metastasis from RCC with lobectomy. The patient survived 23 years.[49] Since this time, not only surgical treatment has changed but medical treatment and radiotherapy have also been modified. In addition to surgery, it has to be evaluated whether adjuvant therapy should be performed or if some patients benefit from systemic therapy only, whether in form of antibodies or, in rare cases, chemotherapy. As stated in the introduction, radiotherapy, especially stereotactic radiation, can derive an advantage for some patients. However, complete resection of lung metastases in selected patients is the therapy of choice to achieve good long-term survival and cure.[6,39,50]

Regarding overall survival, there is no significant difference between the publications released before the year 2000 and after the year 2000. The 5-year survival rate for the publications before 2000 ranged between 32% and 60%, and the median survival ranged between 25 and 39 months[6,7,50-53] (**Table 3**). The literature published after 2000 showed 5-year survival rates between 37% and 49%, with a median survival between 43 and 57 months[37,39-41,48,54,55] (**Table 4**). It can be concluded that the overall

---

Table 3
Publications of pulmonary metastasectomy from RCC before 2000

Author, Year	Overall Survival (5- Year Survival [%]; Median Survival)	Prognosticators
Pogrebniak et al,[51] 1992	60; 43 mo	R0
Cerfolio et al,[52] 1994	36; 36 mo	≥2met, DFI
Vogt-Moykopf et al,[7] 1994	32; 26 mo	DFI, >5
Fourquier et al,[53] 1997	25 mo	N2
Friedel et al,[50] 1999	39; 34 mo	DFI, ≥2 met

Abbreviations: met, metastases; N2, N2 lymph node position; R0, complete resection; size, size of metastasis.

Table 4
Publications of pulmonary metastasectomy from RCC after 2000

Author, Year	Overall Survival (5- Year Survival [%]; Median Survival)	Prognosticators
Pfannschmidt et al,[54] 2002	37	DFI, R0, LNM, $\geq$7 met
Murthy et al,[55] 2005	31	DFI, R0, size, LNM, FEV1$\downarrow$
Hofmann et al,[41] 2005	33; 39 mo	R0, sync, groups
Winter et al,[48] 2010	62 (for R0)	LNM, primary LNM
Kanzaki et al,[40] 2011	47	DFI, R0
Meimarakis et al,[39] 2011	45; 43 mo	R0, size, >3 mets, N2, sync, primary LNM, pleural infiltration, groups
Kudelin et al,[37] 2013	49; 57 mo	Age $\geq$70
Renaud et al,[56] 2014	58; 94 mo	DFI, LNM

Abbreviations: groups, risk groups; met, metastases; N2, N2 lymph node position; R0, complete resection; size, size of metastasis; sync, synchronous.

survival did not improve despite the development of new therapies. Before 2000, fewer patients received operations. With the establishment of metastasectomy, the number of patients with different metastatic patterns increased, but the results did not get worse. Nevertheless, a neoadjuvant or adjuvant treatment must be evaluated for every patient by an interdisciplinary tumor board.

Furthermore, a respectable long-term survival can also be achieved by repeat resection of recurrent metastasis, which is comparable with one-time resection.[39,52,53]

PROGNOSTIC FACTORS OF SURVIVAL

As with other tumor entities, prognostic factors help to select patients. In consideration of prognosticators, the recommendation for metastasectomy can be made by an interdisciplinary tumor board.

Resectability of all metastases is required for recommending a metastasectomy.[7] Incomplete resection is should be considered a contraindication to resection and a negative prognostic indicator. The 5-year survival rates for complete resection are 40% to 50% and for incomplete resection 0% to 22%.[39–41,51,54,55]

The number of metastases also plays a role in metastases of RCC and is debated in the literature.[7,37,39,41,50–52,54] Nevertheless, most of the studies show a significant survival advantage for patients with fewer metastases: the cutoff lies between 2 and 7 metastases.[7,39,50,52,54] Murthy and colleagues[55] see a relationship between multiple metastases in preoperative CT and incomplete resection.

Another important prognostic factor is the DFI. Most of the studies show that a prolonged DFI is significantly associated with a prolonged long-term survival. The period of DFI varied between 12 and 48 months and is most frequently 24 months.[7,39,40,50,52,54–56] Pogrebniak and colleagues[51] and Hofmann and colleagues[41] could not confirm this in their studies. Some studies show a difference between synchronous and metachronous metastases,[39,41] whereas other studies did not find a difference.[51,53]

The intrathoracic lymph node involvement is also debated. Some authors described lymph node metastases as a negative prognostic factor associated with decreased overall survival.[39,48,54–56] The authors' study investigated patients who had a systematic lymph node dissection. The authors could not find a significant difference for lymph node metastases. There was a median survival for patients without lymph node involvement of 72 months, with hilar lymph node involvement of 51 months and mediastinal involvement of 36 months ($P = .232$). This shows that, even with lymph node metastases, a promising long-term survival is reachable.[37] However, other studies did not find a significant influence on survival for lymph node metastases.[7,53] Renaud and colleagues[56] did not find a difference between hilar and mediastinal lymph node metastases.

In addition to influencing factors related to the metastases, factors of the primary tumor seem to influence survival after the resection of metastases. Our data showed a significant difference for the lymph node status and grading of the primary tumor.[38] Two more studies also described a difference for the lymph node status.[39,48] Furthermore, Meimarakis and colleagues[39] find a difference for the size of the primary tumor, whereas we couldn't find an influence for the T status.[38]

PROGNOSTIC GROUPS

Apart from several prognosticators, it is important to investigate prognostic groups that might benefit from metastasectomy. The international registry of lung metastases already published prognostic groups for surgery of metastases in 1997. They divided their patients into 4 groups:

Group 1: Resectable, no risk factors (DFI ≥36 months and single metastasis)
Group 2: Resectable, 1 risk factor (DFI <36 months or multiple metastases)
Group 3: Resectable, 2 risk factors (DFI <36 months and multiple metastases)
Group 4: Unresectable

Using this division, they could show a significant difference in survival for different tumor entities.[57] Here, prognostic factors of different tumor histologies were investigated at the same time. Through this study, justification was given for surgery of metastases.

Following this model, Hofmann and colleagues[41] investigated their patients with metastases of RCC. They found a significant difference in overall survival. Group 1 had a 5-year survival rate of 53%, group 2 48%, group 3 22%, and Group 4 0%.

Because Meimarakis and colleagues[39] only found a difference between the first 3 groups in relationship to the fourth group and not among each other, they developed a new score (Munich score) (**Table 5**).

Risk factors include pleural infiltration, synchronous manifestation of primary RCC and pulmonary metastases, nodal status of the primary tumor, metastasis size greater than 3 cm, mediastinal or hilar lymph node metastases, and completeness of metastasectomy.[39]

These 3 studies show that, using prognostic groups and risk factors, it is easy and fast to evaluate patients for an operation. Of course, other factors like constitution of the patient play a role. An individual selection for each patient should be made despite all prognosticators.

Table 5 Munich Score	
Score	**5-Year Survival**
I (low risk): R0, no risk factor	63%
II (intermediate risk): R0, ≥1 risk factor	29%
III (high risk): R1 or R2 resection	0%[39]

LYMPH NODE DISSECTION AT LUNG METASTASECTOMY FOR RENAL CELL CANCER

RCC can metastasize hematogenously or lymphatically into the thorax (see **Fig. 2**).[37,58,59] The appearance of lymph node metastases, especially from RCC, because of its location, is of particular importance (see **Fig. 1**). The prevalence is described between 26% and 47%.[6,37,39,48,56,60] Nonetheless, only 13% of thoracic surgeons in Europe perform a complete systematic lymph node dissection at metastasectomy.[61] This approach is criticized by some investigators (**Figs. 3** and **4**).[37,39,48,56,60,62]

Dominguez-Ventura and Nichols[62] conclude in their article 5 reasons why a systematic lymph node dissection should be performed:

- There is an incidence of lymph node metastases of 15% to 30%.
- Chest CT has shown a 56% false-negative rate in the evaluation of mediastinal lymph nodes before metastasectomy.
- Radiographically detected mediastinal lymphadenopathy did not correlate with lymph node involvement.
- Even patients with only one single pulmonary metastasis can have involved lymph nodes.
- Mediastinal lymphadenectomy has a recognized low mortality and morbidity.

Because of the high prevalence of lymph node metastases, some investigators demand for a complete resection a systematic lymphadenectomy. Further justifications are the staging and, thus the information, for prognosis of the patient and adjustment of adjuvant therapy.[37,39,48,56,60] Winter and colleagues[48] could find, by matched-pair analyses, a possible advantage for lymphadenectomy.

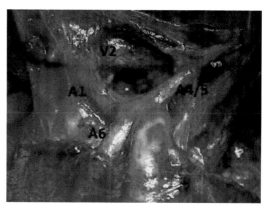

Fig. 3. Interlobar lymph node dissection (right side). A, artery; V, vein.

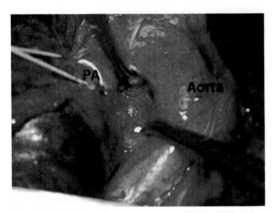

Fig. 4. Mediastinal lymph node dissection (left side). PA, pulmonary artery.

However, Treasure[63] believes that patients with mediastinal lymph node metastases are not curable and, therefore, should be excluded from operation.

The data from this study show that a systematic lymph node dissection can be performed with low morbidity and mortality, and, despite lymph node metastases, a promising long-term survival is attainable (median survival, 37 months). These data also includes patients with lymph node metastases without intrapulmonary metastases. This is a particular phenomenon of RCC.[37]

Because of the high prevalence of lymph node metastases, the complete resection, the staging, the possibility to adjust adjuvant therapy, and the overall good survival for each patient, the authors also request a systematic lymph node dissection in lung metastasectomy of renal cell cancer.

REFERENCES

1. Ferlay J, Soerjomataram I, Ervik M, et al. GLOBO-CAN 2012 v1.0, Cancer incidence and mortality Worldwide: IARC Cancer base No. 11 [Internet]. Lyon (France): International Agency for Research on Cancer; 2013. Available at: http://globocan.iarc.fr. Accessed March 23, 2015.
2. American Cancer Society, Breast cancer survival rates by stage; [Internet]. Available at: http://www.cancer.org/cancer/breastcancer/detailedguide/breast-cancer-survival-by-stage. Accessed March 23, 2015.
3. Coleman RE, Rubens RD. The clinical course of bone metastases from breast cancer. Br J Cancer 1987;55(1):61–6.
4. Kennecke H, Yerushalmi R, Woods R, et al. Metastatic behavior of breast cancer subtypes. J Clin Oncol 2010;28(20):3271–7.
5. Mohan A, Ponnusankar S. Newer therapies for the treatment of metastatic breast cancer: a clinical update. Indian J Pharm Sci 2013;75(3):251–61.
6. Schirren J, Muley T, Schneider P, et al. Chirurgische Therapie der Lungenmetastasen. In: Drings P, Vogt-Moykopf I, editors. Thoraxtumoren, Diagnostik - Staging -gegenwärtiges Therapiekonzept. 2nd Aufl. Heidelberg (Germany): Springer; 1998. p. 640–69.
7. Vogt-Moykopf I, Krysa S, Bülzebruck H, et al. Surgery for pulmonary metastases. The Heidelberg experience. Chest Surg Clin N Am 1994; 4(1):85–112.
8. Senkus E, Kyriakides S, Penault-Llorca F, et al, ESMO guidelines working group. Primary breast cancer: ESMO clinical practice guidelines for diagnosis, treatment and follow-up. Ann Oncol 2013; 24(Suppl 6):vi7–23.
9. Singletary SE, Walsh G, Vauthey JN, et al. A role for curative surgery in the treatment of selected patients with metastatic breast cancer. Oncologist 2003;8(3): 241–51.
10. Rau B, Kandioler D, Stamatis G. Lungenmetastasen. In: Gnant M, Schlag PM, editors. Chirurgische Onkologie Strategien und Standards für die Praxis. 1st Aufl. Wien: Springer; 2008. p. 133–43.
11. Rosen EL, Eubank WB, Mankoff DA. FDG PET, PET/CT and breast cancer imaging. Radiographics 2007; 27(Suppl 1):S215–29.
12. Schirren J, Muley T, Trainer S, et al. Chirurgische Therapie von Lungenmetastasen. In: Schmoll HJ, Höffken K, Possinger K, editors. Kompendium Internistische Onkologie. 4th Aufl. Heidelberg (Germany): Springer Verlag; 2006. p. 958–93.
13. Cerfolio RJ, McCarty T, Bryant AS. Non-imaged pulmonary nodules discovered during thoracotomy for metastasectomy by lung palpation. Eur J Cardiothorac Surg 2009;35(5):786–91 [discussion: 791].
14. Cahan WG, Castro EB. Significance of a solitary lung shadow in patients with breast cancer. Ann Surg 1975;181(2):137–43.
15. Bergmann T, Bölükbas S, Bequiri S, et al. Der solitäre Lungenrundherd Bewertung und Therapie. Chirurg 2007;78:687–97.
16. Welter S, Jacobs J, Krbek T, et al. Pulmonary metastases of breast cancer. When is resection indicated? Eur J Cardiothorac Surg 2008;34(6): 1228–34.
17. Röpke E. Mehrjährige Heilung nach Resektion eines Lungenkarzinoms. Zentralbl f Chir 1937;64:803–6.
18. Yoshimoto M, Tada K, Nishimura S, et al. Favourable long-term results after surgical removal of lung metastases of breast cancer. Breast Cancer Res Treat 2008;110(3):485–91.
19. Lanza LA, Natarajan G, Roth JA, et al. Long-term survival after resection of pulmonary metastases from carcinoma of the breast. Ann Thorac Surg 1992;54(2):244–7 [discussion: 248].

20. Staren ED, Salerno C, Rongione A, et al. Pulmonary resection for metastatic breast cancer. Arch Surg 1992;127(11):1282–4.

21. McDonald ML, Deschamps C, Ilstrup DM, et al. Pulmonary resection for metastatic breast cancer. Ann Thorac Surg 1994;58(6):1599–602.

22. Simpson R, Kennedy C, Carmalt H, et al. Pulmonary resection for metastatic breast cancer. Aust N Z J Surg 1997;67(10):717–9.

23. Friedel G, Pastorino U, Ginsberg RJ, et al. Results of lung metastasectomy from breast cancer: prognostic criteria on the basis of 467 cases of the International Registry of Lung Metastases. Eur J Cardiothorac Surg 2002;22(3):335–44.

24. Ludwig C, Stoelben E, Hasse J. Disease-free survival after resection of lung metastases in patients with breast cancer. Eur J Surg Oncol 2003;29(6):532–5.

25. Planchard D, Soria JC, Michiels S, et al. Uncertain benefit from surgery in patients with lung metastases from breast carcinoma. Cancer 2004;100(1):28–35.

26. Tanaka F, Li M, Hanaoka N, et al. Surgery for pulmonary nodules in breast cancer patients. Ann Thorac Surg 2005;79(5):1711–4 [discussion: 1714–5].

27. Chen F, Fujinaga T, Sato K, et al. Clinical features of surgical resection for pulmonary metastasis from breast cancer. Eur J Surg Oncol 2009;35(4):393–7.

28. Meimarakis G, Rüttinger D, Stemmler J, et al. Prolonged overall survival after pulmonary metastasectomy in patients with breast cancer. Ann Thorac Surg 2013;95(4):1170–80.

29. Yhim HY, Han SW, Oh DY, et al. Prognostic factors for recurrent breast cancer patients with an isolated, limited number of lung metastases and implications for pulmonary metastasectomy. Cancer 2010;116(12):2890–901.

30. Amir E, Ooi WS, Simmons C, et al. Discordance between receptor status in primary and metastatic breast cancer: an exploratory study of bone and bone marrow biopsies. Clin Oncol (R Coll Radiol) 2008;20(10):763–8.

31. World Cancer Research Fund International, Kidney cancer statistics [Internet]. Available at: http://www.wcrf.org/int/cancer-facts-figures/data-specific-cancers/kidney-cancer-statistics#BOTH. Accessed April 3, 2015.

32. Motzer RJ, Bander NH, Nanus DM. Renal-cell carcinoma. N Engl J Med 1996;335(12):865–75.

33. Alt AL, Boorjian SA, Lohse CM, et al. Survival after complete surgical resection of multiple metastases from renal cell carcinoma. Cancer 2011;117(13):2873–82.

34. Oddsson SJ, Hardarson S, Petursdottir V, et al. Synchronous pulmonary metastases from renal cell carcinoma–a whole nation study on prevalence and potential resectability. Scand J Surg 2012;101(3):160–5.

35. Wolchok JD, Motzer RJ. Management of renal cell carcinoma. Oncology (Williston Park) 2000;14(1):29–34 [discussion: 34-6, 39].

36. Motzer RJ, Hutson TE, Tomczak P, et al. Sunitinib versus interferon alfa in metastatic renal-cell carcinoma. N Engl J Med 2007;356(2):115–24.

37. Kudelin N, Bölükbas S, Eberlein M, et al. Metastasectomy with standardized lymph node dissection for metastatic renal cell carcinoma: an 11-year single-center experience. Ann Thorac Surg 2013;96(1):265–70 [discussion: 270–1].

38. Bölükbas S, Kudelin N, Eberlein M, et al. The influence of the primary tumor on the long-term results of pulmonary metastasectomy for metastatic renal cell carcinoma. Thorac Cardiovasc Surg 2012;60(6):390–7.

39. Meimarakis G, Angele M, Staehler M, et al. Evaluation of a new prognostic score (Munich score) to predict long-term survival after resection of pulmonaryrenal cell carcinoma metastases. Am J Surg 2011;202(2):158–67.

40. Kanzaki R, Higashiyama M, Fujiwara A, et al. Long-term results of surgical resection for pulmonary metastasis from renal cell carcinoma: a 25-year single-institution experience. Eur J Cardiothorac Surg 2011;39(2):167–72.

41. Hofmann HS, Neef H, Krohe K, et al. Prognostic factors and survival after pulmonary resection of metastatic renal cell carcinoma. Eur Urol 2005;48(1):77–81 [discussion: 81–2].

42. Wersäll PJ, Blomgren H, Lax I, et al. Extracranial stereotactic radiotherapy for primary and metastatic renal cell carcinoma. Radiother Oncol 2005;77(1):88–95.

43. Motzer RJ, Jonasch E, Agarwal N, et al. Kidney cancer, version 3.2015. J Natl Compr Canc Netw 2015;13(2):151–9.

44. Nirmal TJ, Kekre NS. Management of urological malignancies: has positron emission tomography/computed tomography made a difference? Indian J Urol 2015;31(1):22–7.

45. Park JW, Jo MK, Lee HM. Significance of 18F-fluorodeoxyglucose positron-emission tomography/computed tomography for the postoperative surveillance of advanced renal cell carcinoma. BJU Int 2009;103(5):615–9.

46. Pastorino U, Veronesi G, Landoni C, et al. Fluorodeoxyglucose positron emission tomography improves preoperative staging of resectable lung metastasis. J Thorac Cardiovasc Surg 2003;126(6):1906–10.

47. Farnebo J, Grybäck P, Harmenberg U, et al. Volumetric FDG-PET predicts overall and progression-free survival after 14 days of targeted therapy in metastaticrenal cell carcinoma. BMC Cancer 2014;14:408.

48. Winter H, Meimarakis G, Angele MK, et al. Tumor infiltrated hilar and mediastinal lymph nodes are an independent prognostic factor for decreased survival after pulmonary metastasectomy in patients with renal cell carcinoma. J Urol 2010;184(5):1888–94.

49. Barney JD, Chruchill EJ. Adenocarcinoma of the kidney with metastasis to the lung: cured by nephrectomy and lobectomy. J Urol 1939;42:269–76.

50. Friedel G, Hürtgen M, Penzenstadler M, et al. Resection of pulmonary metastases from renal cell carcinoma. Anticancer Res 1999;19(2C):1593–6.

51. Pogrebniak HW, Haas G, Linehan WM, et al. Renal cell carcinoma: resection of solitary and multiple metastases. Ann Thorac Surg 1992;54(1):33–8.

52. Cerfolio RJ, Allen MS, Deschamps C, et al. Pulmonary resection of metastatic renal cell carcinoma. Ann Thorac Surg 1994;57(2):339–44.

53. Fourquier P, Regnard JF, Rea S, et al. Lung metastases of renal cell carcinoma: results of surgical resection. Eur J Cardiothorac Surg 1997;11(1):17–21.

54. Pfannschmidt J, Hoffmann H, Muley T, et al. Prognostic factors for survival after pulmonary resection of metastatic renal cell carcinoma. Ann Thorac Surg 2002;74(5):1653–7.

55. Murthy SC, Kim K, Rice TW, et al. Can we predict long-term survival after pulmonary metastasectomy for renal cell carcinoma? Ann Thorac Surg 2005; 79(3):996–1003.

56. Renaud S, Falcoz PE, Alifano M, et al. Systematic lymph node dissection in lung metastasectomy of renal cell carcinoma: an 18 years of experience. J Surg Oncol 2014;109(8):823–9.

57. Pastorino U, Buyse M, Friedel G, et al. International Registry of Lung Metastases. Long-term results of lung metastasectomy: prognostic analyses based on 5206 cases. J Thorac Cardiovasc Surg 1997; 113(1):37–49.

58. Reinke RT, Higgins CB, Niwayama G, et al. Bilateral pulmonary hilar lymphadenopathy. An unusual manifestation of metastatic renal cell carcinoma. Radiology 1976;121(1):49–53.

59. Riquet M, Hidden G, Debesse B. Direct lymphatic drainage of lung segments to the mediastinal nodes. An anatomic study on 260 adults. J Thorac Cardiovasc Surg 1989;97(4):623–32.

60. Renaud S, Falcoz PE, Olland A, et al. Should mediastinal lymphadenectomy be performed during lung metastasectomy of renal cell carcinoma? Interact Cardiovasc Thorac Surg 2013;16(4):525–8.

61. Internullo E, Cassivi SD, Van Raemdonck D, et al, ESTS Pulmonary Metastasectomy Working Group. Pulmonary metastasectomy: a survey of current practice amongst members of the European Society of Thoracic Surgeons. J Thorac Oncol 2008;3(11): 1257–66.

62. Dominguez-Ventura A, Nichols FC 3rd. Lymphadenectomy in metastasectomy. Thorac Surg Clin 2006;16(2):139–43.

63. Treasure T. Editorial comment: surgical resection of pulmonary metastases. Eur J Cardiothorac Surg 2007;32(2):354–5.

Thoracoscopic Lung Suffusion

Todd L. Demmy, MD

KEYWORDS

- Regional chemotherapy • Pulmonary suffusion • Isolated lung perfusion • Lung cancer
- Minimally invasive surgery

KEY POINTS

- Compared with strategies targeting other anatomic regions, the popularity of directed lung chemotherapy techniques has been limited most by susceptibility of the lung to direct or indirect injuries of targeted therapy.
- Because each lung holds about 5% of the total blood volume, isolation of one pulmonary organ can allow a 20-fold enhancement of the safe intravenous dose of certain passively absorbed compounds.
- Drugs that are actively transported may not benefit from such a strategy.
- Experimentally and clinically, there seems to be an effect on draining lymph node basins.
- A phase I trial isolating cisplatin for 30 minutes to the side of metastasectomy or primary lung cancer with oligometastases is underway.

 Videos of basic setup and vein isolation, retrograde suffusion flow, and the suffusion sequence accompany this article at http://www.thoracic.theclinics.com/

INTRODUCTION
Burden of Pulmonary Metastatic Disease

In 2015, new US lung cancer cases are predicted to total 221,200, yielding 158,040 deaths, making it the second most common malignancy for both sexes and the most likely cause of cancer-related death.[1] About two-thirds of patients present with an advanced stage requiring chemotherapy for a substantial amount of regional intrathoracic and systemic disease. Even early-stage patients treated solely by surgery or other therapies with the intent of cure will have local recurrence or new tumor develop in their residual lung tissue. Finally, 20% of patients who die from other cancers have the lung as the only disease site, and many malignancies achieve long-term disease control by metastasectomy in about 40% of cases.[2] Any of these situations with locally extensive measurable disease or occult microscopic disease might benefit from a boost of regional chemotherapy or other therapeutic agents if they could be accomplished with minimal risk.

Brief Overview of Suffusion

Thoracoscopic isolated lung suffusion was applied with the goal of achieving practical, safe, regional delivery of pharmacologic or biologic agents. The term *suffusion* describes the diffuse permeation of the lung by injectate during arterial (interventional radiologic) and venous (thoracoscopic) occlusion.[3] This term distinguishes it from infusion methods in which the lack of vascular control limits dose concentration. Alternatively, perfusion techniques recirculate high concentrations of drugs using pumps but require thoracotomy incisions for

Disclosures: There are no relationships to disclose.
Funding: None.
Rutgers Cancer Institute of New Jersey, 195 Little Albany Street, New Brunswick, NJ 08903, USA
E-mail address: todd.demmy@cinj.rutgers.edu

Thorac Surg Clin 26 (2016) 109–121
http://dx.doi.org/10.1016/j.thorsurg.2015.09.013
1547-4127/16/$ – see front matter © 2016 Published by Elsevier Inc.

control and cannulation of delicate pulmonary vessels and risk toxic chemotherapy leakage into the systemic circulation.[4–6]

Synopsis of Competing Open or Minimally Invasive Options

Because of the wide prevalence of isolated pulmonary disease, many investigators have attempted catheter-based interventions including chemoembolization, directed pulmonary artery infusions, and systemic bronchial artery infusions.[7–9] The latter is particularly relevant to lung suffusion because some central tumors derive most of their blood supply from systemic arteries, which might limit the ability to isolate the pulmonary vasculature.[8] There are also approaches that use pumps to recirculate chemotherapeutic agents, but these have been less popular because of limited efficacy, resultant lung injury, and the surgical trauma to the frail patients who might benefit but have impaired overall survival.[10,11] To reduce pump-related toxicity, techniques to improve lung allograft function by ex vivo perfusion are now being tested in vivo for the purpose of delivering cancer therapies.[12]

Anatomy and Physiology Behind Suffusion

The sinusoidal nature of the cardiac circulation and the technique of retrograde cardioplegia was the inspiration behind lung suffusion. Specifically, one report found that giving a heart cardioplegia from both an antegrade (coronary arterial) and retrograde (coronary sinus) uniformly distributed the solution to the organ.[13] A more detailed description of the pulmonary circulation anatomy and physiology was provided before but the most salient points are the following[14]:

- Its circulation is a low-pressure, high-flow, high compliance system that adapts to complete occlusion of one lung with little increase in vascular resistance.
- Blood paths are more of an open sea than tubular, and the lung has an extensive network of supernumerary vessels than can provide collateral flow when needed.
- Only 1% of the lung flow is from bronchial arteries but can be higher in pathologic states, such as tumors garnering systemic flow.
- Alveolar epithelium is adapted to tolerate hypoxia well by increasing glycolytic activity to maintain adenosine triphosphate levels.

PRECLINICAL WORK SUPPORTING SUFFUSION

The suffusion vascular control method was described in preclinical work using nontoxic tracer compounds and was developed to reduce the complexity and morbidity of earlier work.[6,15,16] Previous experiments found rapid permeation of the lung with 75% of tracer remaining in the lung for 30 minutes (**Fig. 1**).[16] Cisplatin was chosen for treatment because it is a familiar agent with efficacy in lung malignancy and tissue uptake kinetics that would be suitable for 30-minute delivery.

Surgical Access and Control of Pulmonary Vasculature

Nineteen immature beagles (6.5–13.8 kg) underwent isolated lung suffusion. Animals met institutional requirements for humane treatment.

A minithoracotomy rather than thoracoscopy was used, as thoracoscopic control in such a small animal was impractical (**Fig. 2**). Furthermore, a less-invasive method of controlling the circulation was already established previously in a larger canine model.[16] The 3 left pulmonary veins (cephalad, middle, and caudal) were controlled with Silastic vascular tapes (Dow-Corning, Midland, MI). Pulmonary artery (PA) cannulations were direct rather than transvenous. A 22-gauge intravenous catheter was inserted into the left main pulmonary artery through a 6.0 polypropylene purse-string to perform the suffusion.

The left lung was collapsed (draining its blood internally) by selectively ventilating the other lung. The veins were snared, and the pulmonary artery was occluded proximally and aspirated distally before injecting the cisplatin solution (1 mg/mL). During suffusion, the left lung was ventilated to aid pulmonary vasculature distention and lung

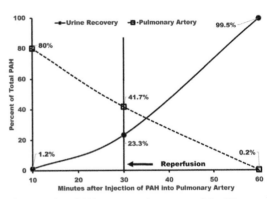

Fig. 1. Urine PAH recovery increases while PA-*para-aminohippurate* (PAH) concentration decreases precipitously after reperfusion, as expected. The urinary recovery before this point is less than 25% of that infused. (*From* Demmy TL, Wagner-Mann C, Allen A. Isolated lung chemotherapeutic infusions for treatment of pulmonary metastases: a pilot study. J Biomed Sci 2002;9:334–8.)

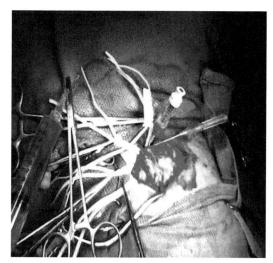

Fig. 2. Immature beagle model (9–10 kg), typically used for preclinical pharmacology toxicity work. Exiting the left anterolateral thoracotomy (head at top and dorsum to right) are silicone tapes snaring the 3 major pulmonary veins and the main left pulmonary artery during suffusion.

permeation. Blood-cisplatin admixture was aspirated from the PA after a 30-minute dwell and then the occlusive bands were released. After reperfusion, the surgical wounds were closed.

Uniform Selective Delivery Experiments

In the first 2 dogs, the left lung was suffused with a systemic dose of cisplatin (2 mg/kg or 40 mg/m^2). Early (first 2 days) toxicities required 50% dose reductions for the second pair of dogs. The fifth dog received a sham operation with saline injection as a control. The suffusate dwelled in the lung for 30 minutes. The left lung underwent biopsy 3 times after suffusion was begun: at 15 minutes (mid-dwell), at 30 minutes (just before reperfusion), and at 60 minutes (washout).

Preclinical Dose Selection Experiments

Suffusion doses were chosen based on the outcomes of the Uniform Selective Delivery component. Each group of 4 received cisplatin suffusions of 0.125 mg/kg, 0.25 mg/kg, or 0.5 mg/kg. Two control dogs were given saline instead.

General Observations

All 19 animals survived the surgical procedure, and 2 were humanely killed before the 30-day endpoint. All 3 saline-control animals recovered uneventfully, and all dogs that survived to the 30-day endpoint maintained baseline cardiac, hematologic, renal, hepatic, and pancreatic function.

Uniform Selective Delivery Experiments

The first 2 full-dose (2 mg/kg) dogs had listlessness, tachypnea, tachycardia, fever, and hemoptysis 24 to 48 hours after the infusion. These symptoms improved by day 5 in dog 1. Dog 2 died on postinfusion day 2. Accordingly, the cisplatin dose was reduced by 50% for the next 2 animals (dogs 3 and 4), and their recoveries were faster.

Dog 1 had a small residual fibrotic left lung 30 days after infusion (**Fig. 3**), whereas dogs 3 and 4 suffered intermediate injuries. Hematoxylin and eosin staining showed evidence of extensive fibrosis corresponding to healing after the toxic injury except in dog 2 that died before these signs of tissue healing could manifest. Dog 1 had 95% parenchymal fibrosis that almost completely replaced blood vessels. Fibrosis was reduced to 40% in dog 3% and 50% in dog 4. Granuloma formation and giant cell accumulation were moderate for all dogs.

Before the start of the dwell (t = 0), there was no measurable platinum in either serum or lung tissue of any dog. Halfway through the dwell (t = 15) and at the conclusion of the dwell (t = 30), platinum was segregated between serum and tissues: mean serum level was 443 ng/mL; mean level in the treated lung was 22,737 ng/g. **Fig. 4** shows the mean tissue levels of platinum from the

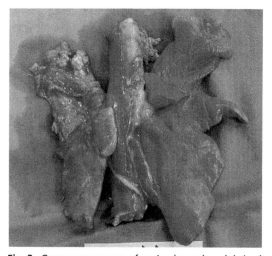

Fig. 3. Gross appearance of canine lungs (caudal view) at necropsy. Specimen from full-dose dog (dog 1) that survived 30 days before elective death. The treated (*left*) side healed leaving a small fibrotic yellow residual lung compared with the normal size pink right side. (*From* Demmy TL, Tomaszewski G, Dy GK, et al. Thoracoscopic organ suffusion for regional lung chemotherapy (preliminary results). Ann Thorac Surg 2009;88:385–90; [discussion: 390–1]; with permission.)

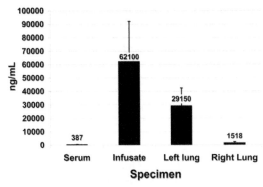

Fig. 4. Cisplatin levels. Relative concentrations (mean) of platinum in various tissues at the end of 30-minute infusion dwell. For the lung tissue specimens, the values are nanograms per gram of tissue.

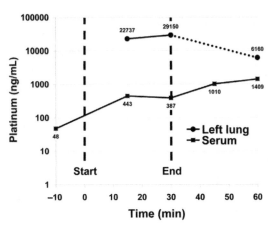

Fig. 5. Platinum washout (logarithmic scale). Graph shows the gradual release of unbound platinum from the treated lung for the high-dose animals during and after the suffusion (starting value compatible with zero platinum given large range required of the assay).

perfused and nonperfused lungs and systemic and perfused pulmonary artery serum just before reperfusion. The data show that the chemotherapy was concentrated in the target lung with little leak to other areas ($P = .01$, one-way analysis of variance). Serum levels increased (**Fig. 5**) to 364%, whereas left lung tissue levels decreased to 21% of the values listed in **Fig. 4** 30 minutes after lung reperfusion.

Preclinical Dose Selection Experiments

Three of the 4 dogs that received 0.5 mg/kg of single lung cisplatin had rapid, raspy, and labored breathing for the first week after infusion. One of them was humanely killed prematurely (day 4) because of lung hemorrhage after intraparenchymal bleeding from a poorly placed PA catheter. The other 2 animals improved by day 10 and had an unremarkable recovery thereafter. Two of the 4 dogs that received 0.25 mg/kg cisplatin were also tachypneic after infusion. However, both improved by day 4, considerably faster than their 0.5-mg/kg counterparts, and had unremarkable recoveries. For the remaining dogs (two 0.25-mg/kg dogs and all 0.125-mg/kg dogs) there were no significant adverse events between infusion and necropsy. **Fig. 6** shows the average number of days it took for the dogs to reach pretreatment eating and respiratory behavior.

The suffused (left) lungs of the dogs that received 0.5 mg/kg and 0.25 mg/kg cisplatin showed fibrosis throughout. In contrast, **Fig. 7** shows the gross and histologic appearance of the lungs from one dog infused with 0.125 mg/kg cisplatin. Like the saline controls, there is no evidence of chemically induced tissue alteration in either lung. **Fig. 8** summarizes the pulmonary and lymphoid histopathologic findings for all 4 dose levels, including the control. There is a general trend toward increased incidence and severity of chronic inflammation and lymphoid atrophy of the paracortex with escalating infusion dose. Accumulation of pigmented macrophages followed the same pattern. Ultimately, draining tracheobronchial lymph nodes showed lymphoid atrophy in 10 of 11 survivors of the low-dose experiments.

Fig. 9 shows the delayed release of cisplatin at the time of reperfusion. As expected, the relationship is dose dependent with a faster falloff for the initial infusate with a higher concentration. The pronounced peak for the highest dose may also indicate tissue saturation had occurred.

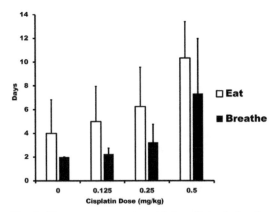

Fig. 6. The average number of days it took for the dogs to eat and return to normal respiration during the recovery period increased in proportion to the infusion dose. Normal respiration was defined by absence of any signs of rapid, raspy, or labored breathing.

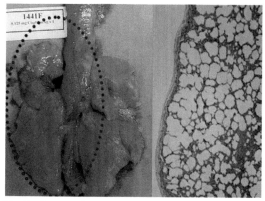

Fig. 7. Gross and histology photographs of one of the dogs that received 0.125 mg/kg cisplatin. Appearance of both lungs are essentially normal, save for areas on the left lung (*circled*) that were adherent to the chest.

SURGICAL TECHNIQUE OF LUNG SUFFUSION

Surgical technique of lung suffusion is depicted diagrammatically in **Fig. 10**.

Preoperative Planning

Currently, patients in our clinical trial are accepted by the inclusion criteria of having cisplatin naïve stage 3 or oligometastatic stage

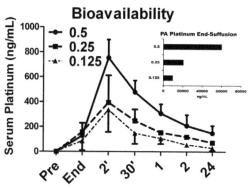

Fig. 9. Delayed release of cisplatin on reperfusion. Time points on x-axis are Pre (preinfusion), End (end of dwell), minutes('), and then hours after reperfusion. Both PA assays and the serum values suggest that once the lung cannot bind any more platinum (beyond 0.25), more is released after suffusion. (*From* Demmy TL, Tomaszewski G, Dy GK, et al. Thoracoscopic organ suffusion for regional lung chemotherapy (preliminary results). Ann Thorac Surg 2009;88:385–90; [discussion: 390–1]; with permission.)

4 lung cancer or pulmonary metastases from other solid organ malignancies. The history, physical examination, and computed tomography (CT) images are reviewed to ensure that the target pulmonary artery can be selectively

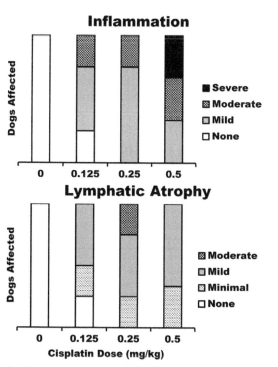

Fig. 8. Proportion of graded pulmonary inflammation and lymphatic atrophy in dogs surviving to day 30 necropsy. The number of animals for the listed dose levels were 2, 4, 4, and 3, respectively.

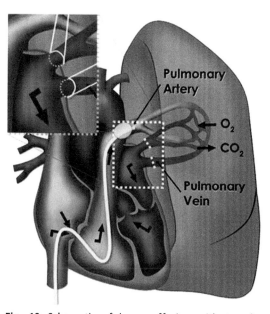

Fig. 10. Schematic of lung suffusion with transfemoral balloon occlusion of left main pulmonary artery and thoracoscopically placed silicone venous snares. (*From* Mallick R, Demmy T. Regional lung chemotherapy techniques. Innovations (Phila) 2011;6:1–9, 3; with permission.)

cannulated, and ipsilateral pulmonary veins can be encircled by video-assisted thoracoscopic surgery (VATS). The patient needs to have sufficient pulmonary reserve to tolerate single lung ventilation and any intended pulmonary resection. The cisplatin dose indicated by the protocol is ordered, and 7.5% of systemic dose (5.62 mg/m^2) is currently the highest dose level completed with acceptable toxicity.

Preparation and Patient Positioning

Patients are prepared and positioned as for any common thoracoscopic procedure. Specifically, patients undergo general endotracheal anesthesia induction by intubation with a double-lumen catheter. The patients are placed in a lateral decubitus position, and the bed is flexed for the vein isolation and lung surgery portions of the operation but is moved back supine for vascular access, fluoroscopy, and lung suffusion. In addition, the patients receive preparatory drugs for the desired chemotherapeutic agent. In these cisplatin cases, they received volume loading with a liter of normal saline and customary antiemetic drugs.

Suffusion Procedure

Isolation of the pulmonary artery and the pulmonary veins proceeded as with the protocol established by the animal model with the difference of performing thoracoscopy with the use of 3 standard lobectomy ports. Through those ports, sublobar or lobar resections and the isolation of the pulmonary vessels can be achieved. Femoral rather than jugular cannulation is the preferred venous access. The main pulmonary artery is occluded by a 9F Arndt bronchial occlusion balloon (Cook Medical, Bloomington, IN) under fluoroscopic guidance (off-label use). This catheter has a tapered low pressure balloon, a central channel large enough to drain the distal pulmonary artery, and a girth that requires placement through a 16F sheath. The remaining protocol is identical to that described above for the animal model and has the following steps.[14]

Vein isolation
The target lung is collapsed by the surgeon's preferred method for single lung ventilation. Using techniques to dissect the veins as if to divide them for thoracoscopic lobectomy, extra long silicone vessel loops (slings) are passed twice to create a snare effect.[17,18] The veins are test occluded. In some cases, a separate middle lobe vein origin or other venous drainage variant requires using more than 2 snares (**Fig. 11**).

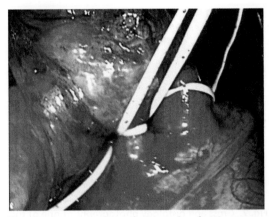

Fig. 11. Intraoperative photograph of vein snares. Separate silicone tapes were required for the middle and upper lobe branches of the superior vein (both exiting from a port near the right upper corner of the photograph. A separate tape around the inferior vein is depicted near the left lower corner.

Ensnarement preparation
The looped snares are laid along the mediastinum within the chest so that they can reach the desired port site without tension even once the lung is re-expanded (Video 1). The loops are secured just beneath the skin of the selected port for later retrieval, and the wound is closed by skin clips or some other temporary method. Ideally, the ports should be placed anterior to the midaxillary line so that they can be accessed easily when the patient is supine for the arterial access procedure. Generally, the most anterosuperior port is used for the superior vein, the more anteroinferior port for inferior vein, and the most inferoposterior port (camera incision) for the chest tube. The lung is then reventilated.

Position change to supine
The wounds are covered sterilely, and the patient is moved from lateral decubitus to supine position (**Fig. 12**). Although it is technically possible to place a PA catheter in the lateral decubitus position, we found this to be difficult and impractical and quickly abandoned it mostly because of the inability to place or ensure proper catheter position throughout the procedure. The advances in operating room imaging, such as the use of hybrid procedure rooms, may change this limitation in the future.

Venous access
With ultrasound guidance and a sterile Seldinger technique, a 16F vascular introduction sheath is introduced into the central venous circulation. The femoral (preferred) or jugular vein (alternate) is used. Patient positioning, preparation, and

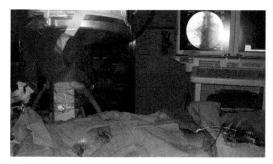

Fig. 12. Adjoining sterile "preps" in patient undergoing right lung suffusion (head and double-lumen at left lower corner of photograph, supine position with slight elevation of right chest to facilitate access to port sites). Two blue silicone tapes (superior and inferior veins) exiting ports beneath the c-arm fluoroscopy image intensifier). An additional, midaxillary, more caudal port with a chest tube is beneath the drape (not visible on photograph). The balloon occlusion catheter sterile field is beneath the fluoroscopy image (*far right*). (*From* Mallick R, Demmy T. Regional lung chemotherapy techniques. Innovations (Phila) 2011;6:1–9, 6; with permission.)

draping (groin or neck) for this portion are done in a way to allow later introduction of a fluoroscopic system and incorporation of the thoracic port sites for the suffusion.

Pulmonary artery occluder placement

Fluoroscopic guidance is used to maneuver a wire/catheter through the right atrium, tricuspid valve, and pulmonary outflow tract into the desired main pulmonary artery. This can be done by a variety of techniques, such as using a flow-directed (Swan-Ganz) catheter, and then exchanging the catheter over a wire. The preference of our interventional radiology team is to use a softer, deflectable tip wire to traverse the pulmonary circulation and then use an exchange catheter to swap the flexible to a stiffer (Amplatz) wire, which is more likely to pass the balloon occluder catheter that has a relatively high durometer. There are several products that contain vascular occlusion balloons that achieve greater than 20 mm size, such as ascending aortic occlusion balloons (Heart-port) used for minimally invasive cardiac surgical operations. We chose to use the Arndt 9 French (Cook Medical, Bloomington, IN, off-label use) bronchial occlusion balloon for several reasons. The catheter has an ideal length and short, low pressure, air-filled balloon engineered to occlude the similarly tapered juxtaposed airway. Although the stiff durometer makes positioning more difficult, it also resists dislodgement once in position. The pulmonary artery anatomy is sufficiently different between patients to warrant development of a

catheter system that achieves a reliable control of vascular inflow without dislodgement or occlusion of side branches, particularly to the upper lobe (**Fig. 13**). Kurenov and colleagues[19] provide a table of PA measurements that might be useful in this regard. Once the catheter is in position, test injections of radiologic contrast ensure flow into upper and lower lobe PA branches during test occlusions of the catheter (see later discussion). A total of 5000 units of heparin are given before the vascular isolation.

Vascular isolation and lung drainage

The Arndt balloon is inflated with air (rather than noncompressible liquids) to reduce risk of artery damage and to allow its visualization by fluoroscopy. This inflation is done just like Swan-Ganz wedge pressure reading by monitoring the PA arterial waveform during inflation until it dampens and decreases to a value consistent with left atrial pressure. The PA pressure is monitored continuously throughout the suffusion to prevent barotrauma or "overwedging" that could induce vascular injury. By this time the previously prepared ports have been exposed, prepared, and draped for surgical access. It is frequently necessary to place a small

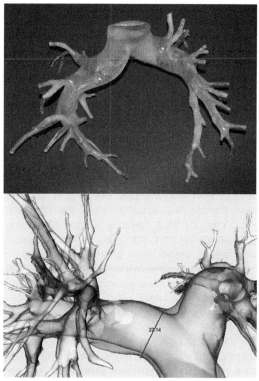

Fig. 13. Pulmonary artery trunk shown by reconstruction of high-resolution CT imaging (*bottom*) and an example of a 3-dimensional printed pulmonary artery (*top*) used to design a better-occlusion catheter.

roll under the ipsilateral chest to make the port more accessible to the surgeon. The fluoroscopy gantry is similarly tilted to maintain the same view used during the PA catheter placement. With the PA occluded, ventilation to the target lung is ceased, and this portion of the airway is drained to facilitate collapse of the target lung yielding internal venous drainage. Next, the vein snares that were retrieved and kept loose are retracted with the same force required to cause occlusion during the VATS portion of the case. Burying the Silastic tapes deep into the jaws of a clamp that is wider than the port incision (bridging the edges of the wound) allows the tension to be maintained. During this lung collapse process, a variable amount of blood (generally 100 to 200 mL) can be withdrawn from the PA catheter port, thus further emptying the PA/venous vascular bed. This process is done by tandem teamwork by the surgeon handing 60-mL syringes to a partner at the venous sheath that immediately reinfuses the blood systemically. Occasionally, PA aspiration may continue beyond that expected, which might represent collateral flow to the lung or some vacuum-related leak around the balloon. As long as the fundamentals of venous occlusion and wedge waveform are seen, the suffusion may proceed.

Lung suffusion
The target lung is inflated and ventilated normally while PA pressures are monitored constantly. When the lung is filled with air, the vascular bed should be relatively empty and eager to accept an infusion from the PA catheter. It is very important not to attempt to infuse the agent before the lung has been ventilated because the vascular bed will be obstructed by the normal physiology that prevents a right-to-left shunt by perfusion of atelectasis. Injecting a small volume of radioactive tracer shows that flow will actually reverse back to the main PA retrograde past the balloon, and the chemotherapy will actually target the opposite lung (Video 2). Thus, injecting a dose of macro-aggregated albumin with Technetium99 tracer immediately before the chemotherapy (same dose used for nuclear medicine perfusion scans) will provide evidence supporting the successful delivery of the suffusate by intraoperative or immediate postoperative scintillation scanning. The chemotherapy is then administered in a small volume (1 mL/kg), compared with the expected 500 mL lung vascular volume, and flushed. The same precautions (extra eye protection, gloves, and special syringe handing) used in the chemotherapy infusion center are followed in the operating room. After administration of the chemotherapy, it dwells for 30 minutes while the PA

pressure is monitored continuously save for brief times that platinum level samples are drawn from the catheter. Even though a small volume of chemotherapy is administered, preclinical work shows that a small amount of radiopaque contrast mixes with innate blood and collateral circulation to suffuse throughout the arterial tree to end up pooling in the obstructed venous system probably facilitated by pressure gradients and the mixing cause by ventilation. Although systemic collateral flow causing vascular overdistention is a theoretic possibility and was seen in some animal experiments in which the PA was controlled by cerclage tape (like the venous side), this has not been observed in our clinical work, possibly because the PA balloon allows for some retrograde decompression. This sequence is shown in the video clip (Video 3).

Suffusion termination
After completion of the suffusion interval, lung perfusion is restored by simply releasing the venous snares and deflating and removing the PA balloon catheter. The snares can be removed by cutting just one side and letting the other side slide out. At this point, with the chest tube already in place, the port wounds can be closed. Alternatively, the lung can be deflated, and the ports can be used to obtain small lung samples for platinum assays and then closed. Patients who require metastasectomy or lobectomy are returned to lateral decubitus position. The venous sheath is removed at the end of the case once the anticoagulant effect of heparin has resolved.

Immediate Postoperative Care

Patients undergo standard postoperative care for a thoracoscopic procedure like a VATS lobectomy and have not required special monitoring or discharge planning. Serum samples for platinum are measured (1) before PA release (at which time samples will be from the isolated pulmonary circulation and systemic circulation) and then (2) 15 minutes and (3) 1 hour from the first draw. PA blood and 2-cm × 2-cm lung samples are obtained approximately 30 minutes after infusion just before control release. If portable scintillation scanning is not available, the patient is sent to nuclear medicine after the procedure to determine whether the radioactive tracer targeted the correct lung (**Fig. 14**). Chest roentgenogram, pulse oximetry, and dyspnea scale at days 2, 3, 7 (each ±1), and 30 (±5) postinfusion are performed. A grade 3 (National Cancer Institute common toxicity criteria)[10] or above nonhematologic toxicity is considered a dose-limiting toxicity if attributed to the isolated lung suffusion procedure.

R   L

Fig. 14. Postsuffusion nuclear medicine (γ camera) imaging shows predominance of technetium macro-aggregated albumin tracer in the target (*left*) lung.

REHABILITATION AND RECOVERY

All patients expected to start their standard advanced-stage chemotherapy (if indicated) uniformly did so within the planned 3 weeks. There are no special discharge instructions or restrictions apart from routine port wound care, and patients return to full activity as tolerated. Evidence of suffusion-related lung dysfunction is investigated by comparing results of functional assessments and objective tests to those before the regional therapy. Six-minute walk tests are used for functional assessments and repeat pulmonary function tests (PFTs) with split lung function assessments are useful. Although the PFT scores may decrease postoperatively from multiple factors such as pain, a relative decrease in the differential perfusion count of the treated lung would be evidence of injury.

CLINICAL RESULTS IN THE LITERATURE
Overview

Thus far, results of lung suffusion have been reported preliminarily from just one center.[3,14] Up to the time of this writing, this procedure has been attempted in 11 patients and was successful in 10. One female patient with metastatic leiomyosarcoma in her lung and liver after multiple operations to resect or ablate her disease had transient mild hypotension and hypoxia of uncertain etiology when snaring the pulmonary veins so the suffusion procedure was aborted. The remaining 10 patients' suffusions (5 right and 5 left) proceeded without incident. Ages ranged from 33 to 73, and 9 patients were women. Thoracoscopic vein control was accomplished reliably in less than 60 minutes, and PA cannulation took less than 30 minutes in all cases except one that was prolonged by attempting to pass the occlusion

catheter transfemorally. In this instance, transient ventricular arrhythmias occurred while attempting to navigate past the right ventricle, and this was the only patient that was observed in intensive care postoperatively. Once the catheter was changed to an internal jugular approach, the occlusion balloon was placed quickly.

All patients were discharged on the first, second or third postoperative days without a major complication or 30-day mortality. Accrual to this study has been slow, not because of a paucity of interested volunteers but the relative expense performing research in the operating room environment (especially for the oligometastatic lung cancer patients that ordinarily would not be offered a surgical procedure). This was less of an issue for metastasectomy cases that are established operations paid by insurance.

Illustrative Cases

The focus of the investigations on this technique has primarily been to determine safety on 2 issues: (1) the ability of patients to tolerate unilateral lung vascular isolations including any injuries that occur attempting vessel control and (2) the ability of the lungs to tolerate the escalating doses of regional chemotherapy.

Complete response of primary, second longest survival (patient 1)

The patient was a 63-year-old woman with a dominant poorly differentiated non–small cell lung cancer of the left lower lobe with a metastatic lesion in the upper lobe and hilar nodes (T2N1M1, American Joint Committee of Cancer, 6th). She underwent a 3.75-mg/m² cisplatin suffusion on February 22, 2008 and was discharged on postoperative day 1. Carboplatin and gemcitabine chemotherapy was scheduled to start on March 5, 2008, and after 2 cycles, there was a significant reduction in the targeted lesions (**Fig. 15**). After 5 cycles from March 23, 2008 to July 2008, the primary lesion had a complete response, but the upper lobe lesion progressed and continued to grow with 2 cycles of pemetrexed (July 2008–September 2008). Weekly docetaxel for 3 months led to disease stabilization until changing to erlotinib (February 2009–April 2009), which was also unsuccessful radiation to the left upper lobe (37.5 Gy, May 14, 2009–June 9, 2009) finally led to disease control for about 4 years until progression required mediastinoscopy and thoracoscopic left upper lobectomy for a yT2N0 tumor. She had no evidence of disease for an additional 7 months until hepatic and bone metastases developed, and she died 72 months from initial therapy.

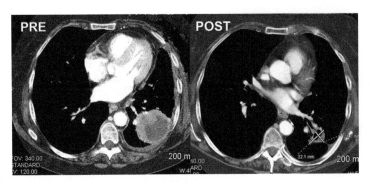

Fig. 15. Case 1 pretreatment (*left*) and 6-week postsuffusion (*right*) CT scan (and after 2 cycles of systemic chemo). Partial response with residual cavity shown. (*From* Demmy TL, Tomaszewski G, Dy GK, et al. Thoracoscopic organ suffusion for regional lung chemotherapy (preliminary results). Ann Thorac Surg 2009;88:385–90; [discussion: 390–1]; with permission.)

Differential response to targeted therapy (patient 4) and longest survival

A 46-year-old woman presented with intractable pain from a C3 cervical metastasis from a right upper lobe adenocarcinoma. There was also a right adrenal metastasis. After palliative radiation to her spine, she underwent 5.625 mg/m^2 cisplatin suffusion on October 31, 2008 and was discharged on postoperative day 1. On November 10, 2008 she began her first dose of cisplatin, docetaxel, and zoledronic acid (Zometa). Just before initiating therapy, the suffused upper lobe tumor had not grown, whereas an adrenal metastasis enlarged significantly (**Fig. 16**). She continued to do well, receiving 4 cycles of chemotherapy with cisplatin, docetaxel, and bevacizumab completed in February 2009 followed by maintenance bevacizumab from February 2009 to April 2012. She then reinitiated chemotherapy with carboplatin and pemetrexed for 2 cycles before and 3 cycles after an adrenalectomy in July 2012 for recurrence (completing treatment in November 2012). She remains alive and disease free now 77 months after suffusion, having recently undergone lumpectomy and radiation for a new primary breast cancer.

Differential response to targeted therapy with failure of systemic therapy (patient 10)

A 70-year-old woman presented with a T4N2M1 squamous cell carcinoma of the right lower lobe complaining of weight loss and abdominal pain with a T6 spinal metastasis. She had a small right upper lobe metastasis, N1 nodes, underwent 5.625 mg/m^2 cisplatin suffusion on October 19, 2011, and was discharged on postoperative day 2. Chemotherapy with carboplatin and gemcitabine began on November 2, 2011. CT imaging only 5 days after initiation of chemotherapy showed reductions in the suffused lung nodule and N1 node but progression of osseous metastases (**Fig. 17**). She achieved some stability in her disease for 8 months but required a craniotomy and whole-brain irradiation for metastatic disease. Her performance status continued to deteriorate, and she died 12 months after suffusion.

Long-term Outcomes of Suffusion Patients

A snapshot of the current outcomes of the lung suffusion program at Roswell Park Cancer Institute is displayed in **Table 1**. Most advanced lung

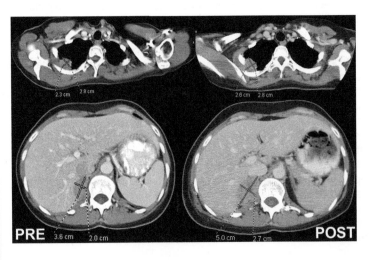

Fig. 16. Case 4 pretreatment (*left*) and postsuffusion (*right*) CT scan (before any systemic therapy). Significant progression of right adrenal metastatic disease is seen with stable or minimally progressive primary disease in the right upper lobe.

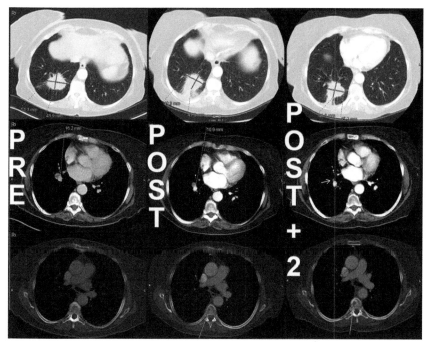

Fig. 17. Case 10 pretreatment (*left*), postsuffusion (*middle*), and post–second cycle (*right*) CT scans. A differential result was observed between primary (stable), suffused N1 nodes (response), and osseous metastases (progression).

cancer patients died, although 2 had prolonged survivals. So far the procedure appears safe from the vascular control standpoint, and there have been no pulmonary toxicities or evidence of reduction in function based on comparing postoperative perfusion imaging with the nontreated side (**Fig. 18**). Although this phase I trial is designed to measure safety, not efficacy, there seems to have been several measureable differences between the behaviors of the suffused lesions compared with the remaining systemic disease. When all lesions respond well, the response could be simply from the overall improvements in the choices and deliveries of chemotherapy observed for lung cancer over the last decade. In these suffusion cases with platinum responsive tumors, the

Table 1
Outcomes from lung suffusion

Case #	Status	Type	Survival (mo)	AE Grades	Outcome
1	Dead	Lung	72	1–3*	CR
2	Dead	Lung	8	1–3*	SD differential effect
3	Dead	Lung	15	1–3*	PR
4	Alive	Lung	59	1–2*	SD differential effect
5	Alive	Sarcoma	64	1–2*	Not evaluable
6	Dead	Lung	9	3	SD differential effect
7	Dead	Lung-BA	23	None	SD
8	Dead	Sarcoma	13	1*	Progression of other sites
9	Alive	Sarcoma	N/A	N/A	Not performed
10	Alive	Lung	14	1*	SD differential effect
11	Alive	Breast	15	1–2*	Not evaluable

Abbreviations: AE, adverse event; BA, bronchoalveolar; CR, complete response; N/A, not applicable; PR, partial response; SD, stable disease.
 * National Cancer Institute Common Terminology Criteria for Adverse Events.

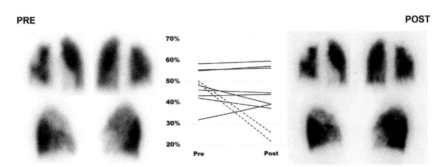

Fig. 18. Split lung function and PFTs before suffusion (Pre) and 6 weeks later (Post). All proportionate function was maintained except for 2 lobectomy cases (*dotted lines*) that decreased to predicted postoperative values.

primary mass essentially gets a head start with treatment (an extra cycle). However, several of the cases had a definite targeted response with progression of systemic disease. Such cases were described in our first clinical report (patient 2), in the case reports above, and in **Table 1**. This phenomenon seems promising given the limited salutary clinical benefits reported for regional lung chemotherapy in the past.

However, it is unknown whether the systemic metastases progress while the suffused areas shrink or remain stable because targeted chemo is more effective than systemic or because of other mechanisms. A cautionary, alternative explanation could be that damaging the primary tumor reduces suppressant cytokines or host immunity, thereby increasing the growth rate of metastases.[20] This negative effect was seen in one young patient with an isolated metastatic malignant peripheral nerve sheath tumor (patient 8) who experienced an eruption of systemic tumor several months after left lung suffusion and concomitant VATS left upper lobectomy. The other metastasectomy patients (suffusion done to control occult minimal residual disease) in this series have done well and are without evidence of disease to date.

SUMMARY

Thus far, minimally invasive regional lung chemotherapy (suffusion) seems to be a safe and reproducible technique to target cancers with disease residing predominately in one lung. There are many potential candidates for this procedure, but accrual has been limited by the high expense of intraoperative research and limited available funding. The somewhat limited benefits shown by previous research using more invasive approaches might have tempered enthusiasm by granting organizations.

Most patients tolerated unilateral lung vascular isolation and then proceeded with lung surgery or definitive chemotherapy without delay. The one step of the clinical procedure that seems to have the greatest potential for failure is the occlusion of the main pulmonary artery with a simple balloon catheter and operator error attempting to suffuse while the lung is collapsed, and the pulmonary vasculature compliance is low. Despite being performed on only a small number of patients, the relative number of differential effects on the targeted tumors is interesting and warrants additional studies using this method. For instance, although nonpathologic lung showed uniform injury in preclinical experiments, it is not known whether tumor or lymphatic vasculature in suffused lungs receives proportionally more or less of the targeted agent. If this work can be reproduced, other agents, like immune modulating compounds, may be more interesting than cytotoxic agents for such regional delivery efforts.

ACKNOWLEDGMENTS

The author acknowledges the invaluable help of Michele Cooper, RN, Garin Tomaszewski, MD, Grace K Dy, MD, Ionnis Platis, MD, John M. Kane III, MD, Jonah H. Patel, Peter Kanter, DVM, PhD, Dongfeng Tan, MD, Thaer Khoury, MD, Lakshmi Pendyala, PhD, and Michael K. Wong, MD toward this research.

SUPPLEMENTARY DATA

Supplementary data related to this article can be found online at http://dx.doi.org/10.1016/j.thorsurg.2015.09.013.

REFERENCES

1. Siegel RL, Miller KD, Jemal A. Cancer statistics, 2015. CA Cancer J Clin 2015;65:5–29.
2. Pfannschmidt J, Egerer G, Bischof M, et al. Surgical intervention for pulmonary metastases. Dtsch Arztebl Int 2012;109:645–51.

3. Demmy TL, Tomaszewski G, Dy GK, et al. Thoracoscopic organ suffusion for regional lung chemotherapy (preliminary results). Ann Thorac Surg 2009;88:385–90 [discussion: 390–1].

4. Grootenboers MJ, Heeren J, van Putte BP, et al. Isolated lung perfusion for pulmonary metastases, a review and work in progress. Perfusion 2006;21: 267–76.

5. Pass HI, Mew DJ, Kranda KC, et al. Isolated lung perfusion with tumor necrosis factor for pulmonary metastases. Ann Thorac Surg 1996;61:1609–17.

6. Weksler B, Burt M. Isolated lung perfusion with antineoplastic agents for pulmonary metastases. Chest Surg Clin N Am 1998;8:157–82.

7. Karakousis CP, Park HC, Sharma SD, et al. Regional chemotherapy via the pulmonary artery for pulmonary metastases. J Surg Oncol 1981;18:249–55.

8. Nakanishi M, Demura Y, Umeda Y, et al. Multi-arterial infusion chemotherapy for non-small cell lung carcinoma–significance of detecting feeding arteries and tumor staining. Lung Cancer 2008;61:227–34.

9. Vogl TJ, Shafinaderi M, Zangos S, et al. Regional chemotherapy of the lung: transpulmonary chemoembolization in malignant lung tumors. Semin Intervent Radiol 2013;30:176–84.

10. den Hengst WA, Hendriks JM, Balduyck B, et al. Phase II multicenter clinical trial of pulmonary metastasectomy and isolated lung perfusion with melphalan in patients with resectable lung metastases. J Thorac Oncol 2014;9:1547–53.

11. Varrassi G, Guadagni S, Ciccozzi A, et al. Hemodynamic variations during thoracic and abdominal stop-flow regional chemotherapy. Eur J Surg Oncol 2004;30:377–83.

12. dos Santos PR, Iskender I, Machuca T, et al. Modified in vivo lung perfusion allows for prolonged perfusion without acute lung injury. J Thorac Cardiovasc Surg 2014;147:774–81 [discussion: 781–2].

13. Carpenter AJ, Follette DM, Sheppard B, et al. Simultaneous antegrade and retrograde reperfusion after cardioplegic arrest for coronary artery bypass. J Card Surg 1999;14:354–8.

14. Mallick R, Demmy T. Regional lung chemotherapy techniques. Innovations (Phila) 2011;6:1–9.

15. Burt ME, Liu D, Abolhoda A, et al. Isolated lung perfusion for patients with unresectable metastases from sarcoma: a phase I trial. Ann Thorac Surg 2000;69:1542–9.

16. Demmy TL, Wagner-Mann C, Allen A. Isolated lung chemotherapeutic infusions for treatment of pulmonary metastases: a pilot study. J Biomed Sci 2002; 9:334–8.

17. Demmy TL, James TA, Swanson SJ, et al. Troubleshooting video-assisted thoracic surgery lobectomy. Ann Thorac Surg 2005;79:1744–52 [discussion: 1753].

18. Watanabe A, Koyanagi T, Nakashima S, et al. How to clamp the main pulmonary artery during video-assisted thoracoscopic surgery lobectomy. Eur J Cardiothorac Surg 2007;31:129–31.

19. Kurenov SN, Ionita C, Sammons D, et al. Three-dimensional printing to facilitate anatomic study, device development, simulation, and planning in thoracic surgery. J Thorac Cardiovasc Surg 2015; 149(4):973–9.e1.

20. Demicheli R, Fornili M, Ambrogi F, et al. Recurrence dynamics for non-small-cell lung cancer: effect of surgery on the development of metastases. J Thorac Oncol 2012;7:723–30.

Index

Note: Page numbers of article titles are in **boldface** type.

A

Ablative approaches for pulmonary metastases, **19–34**
Ablative radiotherapy
  clinical results of, 24–27
  ongoing studies on, 28, 29
  for pulmonary metastases, 23–29
  retrospective studies on, 26, 28
  single-institution studies on, 25
  with systemic therapy, 28
  technical aspects of, 22–24
  toxicity of, 27, 28
Ablative therapies
  and ablative radiotherapy, 23–29
  and microwave ablation, 31
  and oligometastases, 20, 27–31
  principles of, 20, 21
  for pulmonary metastases, 19–31
  and radiofrequency ablation, 29–31
  role of, 20
Adjuvant immunotherapy
  and bacillus Calmette-Guérin, 70, 75
  and bladder cancer, 75
  and breast cancer, 75
  and cancer vaccines, 70–75
  and chimeric antigen-receptor T cells, 70, 73, 74
  and colon cancer, 74, 75
  and cytokines, 70–73
  and interferon, 70–73
  and interleukin-2, 70–73
  and lung cancer, 75
  and melanoma, 70–72
  and programmed death-1, 70–73, 75
  and programmed death ligand-1, 70–73, 75
  and renal cell carcinoma, 72, 73
  and tumor-infiltrating lymphocytes, 70–73, 75
Animal models
  for thoracoscopic lung suffusion, 110–113
Anti-programmed death-1
  and resected pulmonary metastases, 70–73, 75
Anti-programmed death ligand-1
  and resected pulmonary metastases, 70–73, 75

B

Bacillus Calmette-Guérin
  and resected pulmonary metastases, 70, 75
BCG. See *Bacillus Calmette-Guérin.*
BFO. See *Blood flow occlusion.*

The biology of pulmonary metastasis, **1–6**
Bladder cancer
  and adjuvant immunotherapy, 75
Blood flow occlusion
  and isolated lung perfusion, 57
Breast cancer
  and adjuvant immunotherapy, 75
  diagnosis of, 100
  and pulmonary metastasectomy, 99–102

C

CA. See *Cryoablation.*
CAF. See *Cancer-associated fibroblasts.*
Cancer-associated fibroblasts
  and colorectal pulmonary metastasectomy, 45
Cancer vaccines
  and resected pulmonary metastases, 70–75
CAR-T. See *Chimeric antigen-receptor T cells.*
Carcinoembryonic antigen
  and colorectal pulmonary metastasectomy, 43, 44
  and oligometastases, 83, 84, 86
CEA. See *Carcinoembryonic antigen.*
CEA Second-Look trial
  and oligometastases, 84–86
CEASL. See *CEA Second-Look trial.*
Chemotherapeutic agents
  in isolated lung perfusion, 58–64
Chemotherapy
  and isolated lung perfusion, 55–65
  and thoracoscopic lung suffusion, 109–120
Chimeric antigen-receptor T cells
  and resected pulmonary metastases, 70, 73, 74
Cisplatin
  in isolated lung perfusion, 63, 64
  in thoracoscopic lung suffusion, 110–114, 117, 118
Citation network analysis
  and pulmonary metastasectomy, 86, 87
Clamshell thoracotomy
  and pulmonary metastasectomy, 16, 17
Clonality
  of pulmonary metastases, 2
Colon cancer
  and adjuvant immunotherapy, 74, 75
Colorectal carcinoma
  and pulmonary metastasectomy, 41–45, 84–87
Colorectal pulmonary metastasectomy
  and cancer-associated fibroblasts, 45
  and carcinoembryonic antigen, 43, 44

Colorectal (*continued*)
    and disease-free interval, 44, 45
    and KRAS mutations, 45
    and location of metastasis, 44
    and lymph node metastases, 44
    and new prognostic indicators, 45
    and number of metastases, 44
    operative technique for, 42
    and patient selection, 42
    and prognostic factors, 43
    prognostic factors for, 43
    and size of metastasis, 44
    survival outcomes for, 43
Computed tomography
    before pulmonary metastasectomy, 8–10
    before thoracoscopic pulmonary
      metastasectomy, 92, 93, 95, 96
Cryoablation
    for pulmonary metastases, 42, 43
Curative surgery
    and oligometastases, 82, 83
    paradigm of, 79, 80
Cytokines
    and resected pulmonary metastases, 70–73

D

DFI. See *Disease-free intervals.*
Disease-free interval
    and colorectal pulmonary metastasectomy, 44, 45
    and pulmonary metastasectomy, 13–15
    and pulmonary metastasectomy in patients with
      breast cancer, 101, 102
    and pulmonary metastasectomy in patients with
      renal cell carcinoma, 103–105
Doxorubicin
    in isolated lung perfusion, 58

E

EBM. See *Evidence-based medicine.*
ECM. See *Extracellular matrix.*
EGFR. See *Epidermal growth factor receptor.*
ELP. See *Endovascular lung perfusion.*
EMT. See *Epithelial to mesenchymal transition.*
Endovascular blood flow occlusion
    and isolated lung perfusion, 57
Endovascular lung perfusion
    and pulmonary metastases, 63, 64
Ensnarement preparation
    and thoracoscopic lung suffusion, 114
Epidermal growth factor receptor
    and pulmonary metastases, 19, 20, 28
Epithelial to mesenchymal transition
    and pulmonary metastases, 3
Evidence-based medicine
    and pulmonary metastasectomy, 82, 87, 88

Extracellular matrix
    and pulmonary metastases, 3
Extrathoracic metastasis
    and pulmonary metastasectomy, 9, 10
Extravasation
    and pulmonary metastases, 4

F

5-Flurodeoxyuridine
    in isolated lung perfusion, 58–62
FUDR. See *5-Flurodeoxyuridine.*

G

Gemcitabine
    in isolated lung perfusion, 62, 63
Germ cell tumors
    pulmonary metastatectomy for, 51, 52

H

Hemiclamshell thoracotomy
    and pulmonary metastasectomy, 17
HER2 status
    and pulmonary metastasectomy in patients
      with breast cancer, 99, 101, 102
Hyperthermia
    and isolated lung perfusion, 57, 58

I

IFN. See *Interferon.*
IL-2. See *Interleukin-2.*
ILP. See *Isolated lung perfusion.*
Immunity
    in the lung, 69, 70
Immunotherapy for resected pulmonary
    metastases, **69–78**
Interferon
    and resected pulmonary metastases, 70–73
Interleukin-2
    and resected pulmonary metastases, 70–73
Is surgery warranted for oligometastatic disease?,
    79–90
Isolated lung perfusion
    antegrade vs. retrograde, 57
    blood flow occlusion technique for, 57
    chemotherapeutic agents in, 58–64
    and chemotherapy, 55–65
    circuit for, 56
    with cisplatin, 63, 64
    clinical outcomes of, 58–64
    complications of, 64, 65
    and delayed clamp release, 57
    and direct lung injury, 64
    with doxorubicin, 58

endovascular blood flow occlusion technique
for, 57
with 5-flurodeoxyuridine, 58–62
with gemcitabine, 62, 63
and heterogeneous drug distribution, 65
and hyperthermia, 57, 58
and lung to tumor drug concentration, 65
with melphalan, 62
with paclitaxel, 62
and selective pulmonary artery perfusion, 57
surgical techniques for, 56–58
and systemic toxicity, 64, 65
with tumor necrosis factor-α, 62
video-assisted transcatheter, 58
Isolated lung perfusion for pulmonary metastases,
55–67

K

KRAS mutations
and colorectal pulmonary metastasectomy, 45

L

Lung
immune system in, 69, 70
Lung cancer
and adjuvant immunotherapy, 75
and thoracoscopic lung suffusion, 109, 113,
117, 119
vs. metastasis breast cancer, 100
Lung drainage
and thoracoscopic lung suffusion, 115, 116
Lung injury
and isolated lung perfusion, 64
Lymph node dissection
during pulmonary metastasectomy, 105, 106
Lymph node metastases
and colorectal pulmonary metastasectomy, 44
Lymph node sampling
vs. lymphadenectomy during pulmonary
metastasectomy, 36–38
Lymphadenectomy
and pulmonary metastasectomy in patients with
renal cell carcinoma, 105
Lymphadenectomy during pulmonary
metastasectomy, **35–40**
incidence of, 35–37
lymph node sampling vs., 36–38
and prognosis, 38, 39
and survival rates, 39
therapeutic implications of, 39

M

Median sternotomy
and pulmonary metastasectomy, 16

Mediastinal staging
and pulmonary metastasectomy, 8
Melanoma
and adjuvant immunotherapy, 70–72
Melphalan
in isolated lung perfusion, 62
Metastasis
pulmonary, 1–4
Metastasis breast cancer
vs. lung cancer, 100
Microwave ablation
for pulmonary metastases, 31, 42, 43
Minimally invasive surgery
and thoracoscopic lung suffusion, 109–120
and thoracoscopic pulmonary metastasectomy,
91, 92, 95
Munich score
and pulmonary metastasectomy in patients with
renal cell carcinoma, 105
MWA. See *Microwave ablation.*

N

Nonseminomatous germ cell tumors
pulmonary metastatectomy for, 51, 52
NSGCT. See *Nonseminomatous germ cell tumors.*

O

Oligometastases
and ablative therapies, 20, 27–31
and carcinoembryonic antigen, 83, 84, 86
and CEA Second-Look trial, 84–86
and curative surgery, 82, 83
definition of, 80–82
and palliative surgery, 82
and paradigm of curative cancer surgery, 79, 80
and positron emission tomography, 81, 88
and pulmonary metastasectomy, 79–88
and surgery to improve survival, 83
and survival attributed to metastasectomy, 83, 84
Open surgical approaches for pulmonary
metastasectomy, **13–18**
Organ microenvironment
and pulmonary metastases, 4

P

Paclitaxel
in isolated lung perfusion, 62
Palliative surgery
and oligometastases, 82
Patient positioning
for thoracoscopic lung suffusion, 114
for thoracoscopic pulmonary metastasectomy, 93
PD-1. See *Programmed death-1.*
PD-L1. See *Programmed death ligand-1.*

PET. See *Positron emission tomography.*
Positron emission tomography
  and oligometastases, 81, 88
  before pulmonary metastasectomy, 8, 9
Posterolateral thoracotomy
  and pulmonary metastasectomy, 16, 17
Preclinical dose selection experiments
  and thoracoscopic lung suffusion, 111, 112
Preoperative evaluation and indications for
  pulmonary metastasectomy, **7–12**
Primary malignancy
  and pulmonary metastasectomy, 9, 10
Programmed death-1
  and resected pulmonary metastases, 70–73, 75
Programmed death ligand-1
  and resected pulmonary metastases, 70–73, 75
Pulmonary artery occluder
  and thoracoscopic lung suffusion, 115
Pulmonary function testing
  and pulmonary metastasectomy, 8, 9
Pulmonary metastasectomy
  and breast cancer, 99–102
  and citation network analysis, 86, 87
  and clamshell thoracotomy, 16, 17
  and colorectal carcinoma, 41–45, 84–87
  and control of extrathoracic metastasis, 10
  and control of primary malignancy, 9, 10
  and CT preoperative evaluation, 8–10
  and disease-free intervals, 13–15
  and evidence-based medicine, 82, 87, 88
  and extended incisions, 16, 17
  and extrathoracic metastasis, 9, 10
  future of, 87, 88
  and hemiclamshell thoracotomy, 17
  indications for, 9–11
  lymphadenectomy during, 35–40
  and median sternotomy, 16
  and mediastinal staging, 8
  and muscle-sparing incisions, 16
  and oligometastases, 79–88
  open surgical approaches for, 13–17
  and patient history, 7, 8
  and posterolateral thoracotomy, 15, 16
  preoperative evaluation for, 7–9
  and preoperative imaging, 8
  and preoperative physical examination, 7, 8
  and pulmonary function testing, 8, 9
  and renal cell carcinoma, 102–106
  and sarcoma, 87
  thoracoscopic, 91–96
  and tumor resectability, 10
  unwarranted enthusiasm for, 88
  and video-assisted thoracic surgery, 14, 15
  vs. nonoperative management, 10
Pulmonary metastasectomy in patients with breast
  cancer
  and disease-free interval, 101, 102
  and HER2 status, 99, 101, 102
  and prognostic factors, 101, 102
  and prognostic groups, 102
  reports in the literature of, 101, 102
  role of, 99–102
  and survival, 100, 101
Pulmonary metastasectomy in patients with
  renal cell carcinoma
  and disease-free interval, 103–105
  lymph node dissection during, 105, 106
  and lymphadenectomy, 105
  and Munich score, 105
  and prognostic factors, 104
  and prognostic groups, 105
  reports in the literature of, 103, 104
  and survival, 103, 104
Pulmonary metastases
  ablative approaches for, 19–31
  and ablative radiotherapy, 23–29
  biology of, 1–4
  clonality of, 2
  and colorectal pulmonary metastasectomy, 41–45
  and cryoablation, 42, 43
  and endovascular lung perfusion, 63, 64
  and epidermal growth factor receptor, 19, 20, 28
  and epithelial to mesenchymal transition, 3
  and extracellular matrix, 3
  and extravasation, 4
  heterogeneity of, 2
  hybrid treatment of, 42, 43
  and immunotherapy after resection, 69–75
  and indications for metastasectomy, 9–11
  isolated lung perfusion for, 55–65
  and lymphadenectomy during metastasectomy,
    35–40
  and metastatectomy, 49–53
  and metastatectomy vs. therapeutic options,
    49, 50
  and microwave ablation, 31, 42, 43
  nonoperative treatment of, 42, 43
  and open surgical approaches, 13–17
  and organ microenvironment, 4
  pathogenesis of, 1, 2
  and preoperative evaluation for
    metastasectomy, 7–9
  and radiofrequency ablation, 29–31, 42
  and seed and soil hypothesis, 2–4
  and stereotactic body radiation therapy, 19, 21,
    22, 24, 27–30
  and survival and arrest in transit, 3, 4
  thoracoscopic management of, 91–96
  and tumor cell adherence, 3
  and tumor cell motility, 3
  and video-assisted thoracoscopic surgery, 42
Pulmonary metastatectomy
  complications of, 52
  for germ cell tumors, 51, 52

for nonseminomatous germ cell tumors, 51, 52
and retroperitoneal lymph node dissection, 52
for sarcoma, 50, 51
surgical technique for, 49, 50
Pulmonary metastatic disease
and open vs. minimally invasive surgery, 110
Pulmonary vasculature
and thoracoscopic lung suffusion, 110, 111

R

Radiofrequency ablation
outcomes of, 29–31
for pulmonary metastases, 29–31, 42
technique of, 29
RCC. See Renal cell carcinoma.
Renal cell carcinoma
and adjuvant immunotherapy, 72, 73
diagnosis of, 103
and pulmonary metastasectomy, 102–106
Results of pulmonary resection: Colorectal
carcinoma, **41–47**
Results of pulmonary resection: Other epithelial
malignancies, **99–108**
Results of pulmonary resection: Sarcoma and germ
cell tumors, **49–54**
Retroperitoneal lymph node dissection
and pulmonary metastatectomy, 52
RFA. See Radiofrequency ablation.
RPLND. See Retroperitoneal lymph node dissection.

S

Sarcoma
and adjuvant immunotherapy, 73, 74
and pulmonary metastasectomy, 87
and pulmonary metastatectomy, 50, 51
SBRT. See Stereotactic body radiation therapy.
Seed and soil hypothesis
and pulmonary metastases, 2–4
Selective pulmonary artery perfusion
and pulmonary metastases, 57
SPAP. See Selective pulmonary artery perfusion.
Stereotactic body radiation therapy
and pulmonary metastases, 19, 21, 22,
24, 27–30
Systemic therapy
with ablative radiotherapy, 28

T

Thoracoscopic lung suffusion, **109–121**
anatomy and physiology behind, 110
animal models for, 110–113
and chemotherapy, 109–120
with cisplatin, 110–114, 117, 118
and clinical results in the literature, 117–120

and control of pulmonary vasculature, 110, 111
and ensnarement preparation, 114
and immediate postoperative care, 116, 117
and long-term outcomes, 118–120
and lung cancer, 109, 113, 117, 119
and lung drainage, 115, 116
and minimally invasive surgery, 109–120
overview of, 109, 110
and patient positioning, 114
and preclinical dose selection experiments,
111, 112
preclinical work supporting, 110–113
preoperative planning for, 113, 114
and pulmonary artery occluder placement, 115
and pulmonary metastatic disease, 109
and rehabilitation and recovery, 117
and supine positioning, 114
surgical access for, 110, 111
surgical technique for, 113–116
termination of, 116
and uniform selective delivery experiments,
111, 112
and vascular isolation, 115, 116
and vein isolation, 114
and venous access, 114, 115
and video-assisted thoracoscopic surgery, 114,
116, 120
Thoracoscopic management of pulmonary
metastases, **91–97**
Thoracoscopic pulmonary metastasectomy
and clinical results in the literature, 95, 96
and minimally invasive surgery, 91, 92, 95
patient positioning for, 93
and postoperative course, 94, 95
and preoperative CT scanning, 92, 93, 95, 96
and preoperative planning, 92, 93
surgical technique for, 92–94
and video-assisted thoracic surgery, 92–96
Thoracotomy
clamshell, 16, 17
hemiclamshell, 17
posterolateral, 15, 16
TIL. See Tumor-infiltrating lymphocytes.
TNF-α. See Tumor necrosis factor-α.
Toxicity
of ablative radiotherapy, 27, 28
and isolated lung perfusion, 64, 65
Tumor cells
adherence of, 3
motility of, 3
and survival and arrest in transit, 3, 4
Tumor-infiltrating lymphocytes
and resected pulmonary metastases, 70–73, 75
Tumor necrosis factor-α
in isolated lung perfusion, 62
Tumor resectability
and pulmonary metastasectomy, 10

U

Uniform selective delivery experiments
    and thoracoscopic lung suffusion, 111, 112

V

Vascular isolation
    and thoracoscopic lung suffusion, 115, 116
VATS. See *Video-assisted thoracic surgery.*
Vein isolation
    and thoracoscopic lung suffusion, 114

Venous access
    and thoracoscopic lung suffusion, 114, 115
Video-assisted thoracic surgery
    and pulmonary metastasectomy, 14, 15
    for pulmonary metastases, 42
    and thoracoscopic lung suffusion, 114, 116, 120
    and thoracoscopic pulmonary metastasectomy,
        92–96
Video-assisted transcatheter isolated lung
    perfusion
    and pulmonary metastases, 58

Moving?

Make sure your subscription moves with you!

To notify us of your new address, find your **Clinics Account Number** (located on your mailing label above your name), and contact customer service at:

Email: journalscustomerservice-usa@elsevier.com

800-654-2452 (subscribers in the U.S. & Canada)
314-447-8871 (subscribers outside of the U.S. & Canada)

Fax number: 314-447-8029

Elsevier Health Sciences Division
Subscription Customer Service
3251 Riverport Lane
Maryland Heights, MO 63043

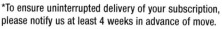

Printed and bound by CPI Group (UK) Ltd, Croydon, CR0 4YY

08/05/2025

01864680-0008